"*Jungian Reflections on Systematic Racism: Members of an American Psychoanalytic Community on Training, Practice, and Inclusivity* is a unique new book co-edited by Jungian Psychoanalysts Christopher Carter and Tiffany Houck, both members of the Jungian Psychoanalytic Association (NY). The brilliant uniqueness of this book is its' stellar light shone on the darkness of the racialized aspects of Jungian training that is seen in print. Bravo! For the courage of the book's authors. This book belongs on the shelf of every psychoanalyst in training and every professional in the field of Psychology."

Dr. Fanny Brewster, *Jungian Analyst, Professor at Pacifica Graduate Instittue, and author of* The Racial Complex: A Jungian Perspective on Culture and Race *(Routledge, 2019)*

"Christopher J. Carter and Tiffany Houck's wonderful book, *Jungian Reflections on Systemic Racism,* provides a container for our potential encounters with Jung's relations to racialized cultural complexes that appear both in his writings and in analytic training institutes. The contributors find that some of C.G. Jung's writings appear to mirror colonial attitudes, a kind of Social Darwinism, even as Jung's writings offer a theory of individuation as a potential. Reflecting upon Jung, this book's contributors make space and give voice to their encounters with the unconcious, exemplifying ways of working with our own racialized complexes."

Samuel Kimbles, PhD, *author of* Intergenerational Complexes in Analytical Psychology: The Suffering of Ghosts *(Routledge, 2021)*

"*Jungian Reflections on Systemic Racism* is a hugely significant and original volume. Based on experiences in Jungian analysis and institutional life, but going beyond that community to embrace all approaches to psychotherapy, it offers a demonstration of how to divest our profession from its role in systemic – and casual – racism. With great frankness, the authors consider individual attitudes, responsibilities, and roles. This is the basis on which they seek to reframe approaches, teachings, and writings on ethnic, cultural and social dimensions of experience in therapy and society."

Andrew Samuels, *author of* The Political Psyche *(Routledge, 2015)* *and* A New Therapy for Politics? *(Routledge, 2015)*

T0384877

Jungian Reflections on Systemic Racism

Jungian Reflections on Systemic Racism is a unique contribution of Jungian analysts and analysts-in-training who provide individual perspectives and approaches to promoting greater inclusivity in analytical theory, training and practice.

This book examines issues of racism through intrapsychic, interpersonal, and archetypal lenses. Drawing from the specificity and ingenuity of Jungian psychoanalysis, the authors provide personal narratives, clinical vignettes, and theoretical perspectives that exemplify ways of comprehending and furthering the work of anti-racism. The editors assert that without deeper exploration of our theories, distinguishing between the theory itself and the theorist's unconscious biases, our clinical paradigms unconsciously align and thus perhaps promote an attitude of white supremacy in psychoanalytic training programs and practices. Without claiming to reflect the official view of any particular psychoanalytic community, it utilizes Jung's analytic paradigm to offer insight into the dynamics of the cultural complex of racism from a depth psychological perspective.

Jungian Reflections on Systemic Racism is an important resource for psychoanalytic students, trainees, supervisors, and practitioners, as well as for clinicians, medical professionals, social workers, mental health professionals, sociologists, and anyone interested in the wide impact of the unscientific construct of 'race'.

Christopher Jerome Carter, MDiv, ThM, PhD, LP, NCPsyA is certified in Jungian analysis and is a licensed psychoanalyst practicing in New York. He is a member of the International Association for Analytical Psychology (IAAP), the National Association for the Advancement of Analytic Psychology (NAAP), and the Jungian Psychoanalytic Association. 'Time for Space at the Table: An African American-Native American analyst-in-training's first-hand reflections. A call for the IAAP to publicly denounce (but not erase) the White supremacist writings of C.G. Jung' was honored with the 2021 Gradiva Award (NAAP).

Tiffany Houck, MDiv, PhD, LP is a licensed psychoanalyst and a certified Jungian analyst in private practice in New York City. She is the author of *History Through Trauma: History and Counter-History in the Hebrew Bible* (2018, Wipf and Stock Publishers); as well as numerous journal articles and book chapters published at the intersection of studies in gender and sexuality, psychoanalysis, religion, and trauma. She serves as a faculty member and the current Director of Training of the Jungian Psychoanalytic Association.

Jungian Reflections on Systemic Racism

Members of an American Psychoanalytic Community on Training, Practice and Inclusivity

Edited by Christopher Jerome Carter and Tiffany Houck

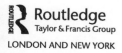

Routledge
Taylor & Francis Group

LONDON AND NEW YORK

Designed cover image: Graciela Vilagudin as rendered the owner on
Getty Images

First published 2023
by Routledge
4 Park Square, Milton Park, Abingdon, Oxon OX14 4RN

and by Routledge
605 Third Avenue, New York, NY 10158

Routledge is an imprint of the Taylor & Francis Group, an informa business

British Library Cataloguing-in-Publication Data
A catalogue record for this book is available from the British Library

Library of Congress Cataloging-in-Publication Data
Names: Carter, Christopher (Christopher Jerome), editor. | Houck, Tiffany,
editor.
Title: Jungian reflections on systemic racism : members of an American
psychoanalytic community on training, practice and inclusivity / edited by
Christopher Carter and Tiffany Houck.
Description: Abingdon, Oxon ; New York, NY : Routledge, 2023. | Includes
bibliographical references and index. |.
Identifiers: LCCN 2022058391 (print) | LCCN 2022058392 (ebook) | ISBN
9781032318035 (paperback) | ISBN 9781032318042 (hardback) | ISBN
9781003311447 (ebook)
Subjects: LCSH: Jungian psychology--Moral and ethical aspects. |
Psychoanalysis--Moral and ethical aspects. | Racism.
Classification: LCC BF173.J85 J895 2023 (print) | LCC BF173.J85 (ebook) |
DDC 150.19/54--dc23/eng/20230415
LC record available at https://lccn.loc.gov/2022058391
LC ebook record available at https://lccn.loc.gov/2022058392

ISBN: 978-1-032-31804-2 (hbk)
ISBN: 978-1-032-31803-5 (pbk)
ISBN: 978-1-003-31144-7 (ebk)

DOI: 10.4324/9781003311447

'We dedicate this volume to the reader and to all healthcare students and professionals seeking to promote wellness through greater inclusivity'

Please be aware that this book contains sensitive language.

Contents

Notes on the Contributors

Ann Ulanov, MDiv, PhD, LHD is a certified Jungian analyst practicing in New York City and Emerita Johnson Professor of Psychology and Religion at Union Theological Seminary (NYC) as well as a member of Jungian Psychoanalytic Association and International Association for Analytical Psychology (IAAP). She is the author of many books. Her most recently published books are *The Psychoid, Soul and Psyche: Piercing Space/Time Barriers* and *Back to Basics*.

Deborah Fausch, PhD, LP is a certified Jungian analyst and licensed psychoanalyst practicing on the East Coast of the United States and in Mexico. Having previously practiced and taught as an architect and architectural historian, she is especially interested in color imagery as a place where culture, history, materiality, subjectivity, and the archetypal engage in concrete and symbolic resonance.

Sherry Salman, PhD, LP is a certified Jungian analyst practicing in upstate New York. A founding member and the first President of the Jungian Psychoanalytic Association, she now serves on the faculty and has contributed to the education of many Jungian analysts and psychotherapists.

Amy Bentley Lamborn, MDiv, PhD is an analyst-in-training at the Jungian Psychoanalytic Association. She is the author of numerous publications, including 'The *Deus Absconditus* and the Post-Secular Quest' in *Jung in the Academy and Beyond*, 'The Fourth/Reduction: Carl Jung, Richard Kearney, and the *Via Tertia* of Otherness' (in *Psychology and the Other*), and a forthcoming book, *Figuring the Self/Figuring the Sacred* (Pickwick Publications). An Episcopal priest and a therapist in private practice, she is also Visiting Professor of Pastoral and Contextual Theology at the School of Theology, University of the South, in Sewanee, Tennessee and is a frequent lecturer on depth psychology and religion.

John Michael Hayes, PhD, ABPP is a psychologist and psychoanalyst in private practice in Baltimore, MD. He is a priest of the Episcopal Diocese of Maryland. He holds faculty appointments in the Department of

Psychiatry at the University of Maryland School of Medicine, the Washington-Baltimore Psychoanalytic Institute, and the Ecumenical Institute of St. Mary's Seminary & University. John is an analyst-in-training at the Jungian Psychoanalytic Association in New York City.

Sarah J. Braun, M.D. is a certified Jungian Psychoanalyst in private practice in Narberth, Pennsylvania. She works primarily with adults, and also with children, teenagers, emerging adults and couples. She is board certified in General Psychiatry as well as Child and Adolescent Psychiatry, and is an analyst member of the Jungian Psychoanalytic Association of New York and the Philadelphia Association of Jungian Analysts of the Philadelphia Jung Institute.

Preface

What follows this perspectival comment, one I am humbled to offer, embodies and invites a shedding of habit, ours. The garments of our daily personal and communal thinking, finely honed and well assembled habits, sadly are identified with our very being. Jungian Psychoanalysis precisely engages this existential geography and its all too familiar ailments.

Each author, Jungian Analysts and Jungian Analysts in Training, whose contributions in toto make up this superb collection, inspired and shepherded by Christopher J. Carter and Tiffany Houck, has been part of an ongoing conversation, a willing shedding and re-garmenting, circling around personal experiences of pejorative othering, as subjects and as personal authors. From this perspective, the maximal generativity of their essays will be reflected in our own taking up the mantle of our own conversations and willingly bearing what they offer to being into birth, new being.

Each essay, additionally, offers a rethinking, a reimagining, a fresh ensoulment, of our prized paradigms of thought and process, of individual and collective change, of psychoanalysis and cultural change. Many roots of thought and action are woven into these offerings: architecture, theology, the many lines of therapeutic process—pastoral care, social work, psychology, psychiatry, mental health counseling, psychoanalysis. Nonetheless, each reflection offers something novel and nourishing, regardless of one's familiarity with any of these fields.

Over the years, in various capacities, I have been privileged to know each contributor, and with each this privilege has yielded unexpected awakenings, such shifting of perspective as we associate with generative mutuality. As you read further in this volume, join me in the liminal space it offers, over and over, as such a journey will suit us all well.

Harry Wells Fogarty

Biographical Note

Harry Wells Fogarty, MDiv, PhD, LP is a Jungian Analyst practicing in NYC, who also serves as a Faculty Member for both the Jungian Psychoanalytic Association of New York and the Philadelphia Association of Jungian Analysts.

Introduction

Christopher Jerome Carter and Tiffany Houck

Christopher Jerome Carter

On 14 July 2019, the Jungian Psychoanalytic Association (JPA, New York City) offered 'Jung & Race', a workshop that preceded the International Association for Analytical Psychology's Vienna conference. I attended, hoping the JPA would acknowledge Jung's imperfection and assimilate analytic theory more inclusively, inviting people who are not white to advance our paradigm.

The workshop introduced participants to *cognitive bias* and explored the impact of unconscious bias on hermeneutics. Readings included 'Open Letter from a group of Jungians on the question of Jung's writings on and theories about "Africans"' (2018), and Farhad Dalal's 'Jung: A racist' (1988). I was invigorated by the Open Letter's call for increased attention to biases against intercultural perspectives to the point of 'correcting and changing theories that harm people of colour'. Having recently read Fanny Brewster (2017), I was uplifted in seeing her name amongst the analysts beckoning change, including Samuel L. Kimbles and Alan G. Vaughan.

The greater impact was made directly within the workshop. I was pleasantly surprised by the facilitators' solidarity with the three participating analysts-in-training (myself included), at an official training event. It was healthful to masticate previous class discussions in which Jung's offences had been treated as irreproachable. I had felt like an imposter in classrooms and in psychoanalytic seminars, even those sponsored by other training institutes. Finally, there was space for me at the table.

On 4 August 2019, Harry Wells Fogarty (who was then JPA's Clinical Evening Coordinator), invited me to participate in JPA's 2019 Fall Colloquium. He suggested that most of the institute's community—though well-intentioned—may be so embedded in white structures that we may be unaware of our lack of openness, and he invited me to address diversity within analytic theory and training structures. I accepted the offer after approaching each participant of the Jung & Race workshop, inviting them to join me. All who attended the class agreed to join in a panel discussion. Following the panel discussion, virtually all participants of our community

DOI: 10.4324/9781003311447-1

approached me. I was dumbfounded by the collective response. Something had shifted, something reportedly long undisclosed in constellation. Following my talk on the panel, Dr. Fogarty nudged me into publishing my talk as an article. He introduced me to Andrew Samuels, who graciously introduced me to the remarkable editors of the *Journal of Analytical Psychology*, Marcus West and Nora Swan-Foster.

As I was writing, the world shifted. As much of the world shut down, there was space for the media to cover what appeared to be an increased rate of egregious murders against Blacks by whites. The video of the murder of George Floyd made this long-standing problem yet more transparent. World-wide, people of varying nations, ethnicities, colors, ages, languages protested in large numbers against the systemic brutality against Blacks, Indians, and People of Color (BIPOC). While we could unite to eradicate COVID-19, we needed to do more work on unmasking and eradicating systemic hatred against people of color and the denial of our inalienable rights as fully human beings. The root of the problem is not only within individuals; it is systemic and too numinous for most to verbalize. I take umbrage with Jung's written attacks against Blacks and North American's First Nations; but the call is not just to effect change amongst Jungians. The medical and mental health professions have played a significant role in institutionalizing the notion of race; so we have a responsibility to re-educate the general population to the invalidity of 'race', the unsubstantiated cornerstone of systematized racism—a potential barrier to greater individuation within us all.

I urged the JPA to make a public statement denouncing race and systematized racism. Many awkward discussions were held by our collective regarding the personal responsibility to the collective, and how to denounce inequality without shutting the door on persons who have conflicting stances on inclusivity. Tiffany Houck showed great empathy, courage, perseverance, and foresight in keeping this subject matter in discussion. To my grateful surprise, so do others. Tiffany's solidarity had existed in our friendship and in her personal journey. Among others, Donald Grasing, then JPA's President and one of my supervising analysts, was also supportive in contemplating the impacts of bias on our learning community and in seeking balance. In the later part of 2021, Routledge offered me the possibility of expanding on my article, 'Time for Space at the Table', into a book. I found this to be a great opportunity for analysts and analysts-in-training to give voice to their experiences and perspectives on the matter of race. Tiffany agreed to be the co-editor, and we approached people who had openly voiced their support for the advancement of our paradigm and for disempowering the construct, race.

Jungian Reflections on Systemic Racism: Members of an American Psychoanalytic Community on Training, Practice, and Inclusivity is a volume of essays contributed by Jungian analysts and analysts-in-training who are part of the Jungian Psychoanalytic Association (New York), a learning community and analytic training institute. We are not the first to write on racism through a psychoanalytic theory. We are greatful to all who have and continue to blaze the trail toward greater tolerance toward the *other*. This volume could not possibly speak to the full history, psychology and collective impact of the "race" lie and the politics and powers that continue its systematization. We enter the conversation in a way that links our personal experiences and reflections, differentiating the individual from the collective in such a distinctly Jungian process that returns us to the collective with fresh perspectives.

Exemplifying attitudes through which psychoanalytic institutes might formally address systematized racism and denounce 'race', the contributors of *Jungian Reflections on Systemic Racism* interrogate problematic aspects within our own paradigm. The contributors respond to aspects of Jung's writings and Jungian theory that reflect attitudes of xenophobia and white supremacy as they work toward increased consciousness of their own racialized ways of perceiving the *other*, of teaching, and of practicing. This volume exemplifies an attitude of appreciating Jung's image as less of a haunting figure than of an ancestor who offers a cautionary tale of the harm that may result from a lack of consciousness in one's 'healing' method and practice. Personal experiences and clinical vignettes serve to exemplify a psychoanalytic method of deconstructing systemic racism within Jungian theory and within analytic practice. While we do not have all of the answers to this complexity, the specificity and ingenuity of C. G. Jung's depth psychological paradigm offers insight into the shadow work of inclusivity.

Jungian Reflections on Systemic Racism may not correspond with the experiences, perspectives, or attitudes of other persons of color, within the JPA, or in other psychoanalytic learning communities. There are Jungians who thrust aside concerns of Jung's racist writings, as if needing to avoid Jung in his wholeness. Not every Jungian idolizes Jung, but many exalt him. Inquisitive analysands ask, 'Did Jung support racism? What is the "analytical attitude" towards systemic racism?' In concealed ways, the psychoanalytic field continues to play a significant role in the systemization of race ideology, which is a false science. *Racism is real. Racists exist. But race does not exist.* We stand by the efficacy and unique benefits of analytic psychology. Jung is not able to defend himself against currently stated complaints. We seek an appreciation of Jung, in a clear-eyed way, to cultivate greater embodiment of the analytic process, nurturing the expansion of analytic theory.

This work is not to be mistaken as polemical. Its 'telos' is neither to present controversy nor to attack a patriarch. This is the right moment for analysis to promote global solidarity, unmasking the gems that reverberate within global tensions. In turning a blind eye:

What we preach we cannot put into practice, for we do not hold the opposites and hear their tension, consciously, thus inhabiting a space between. We sever instead.

(Ulanov 2014, p. 129)

Tiffany Houck

On 26 May 2020, one day after the murder of George Floyd, riots were starting to erupt throughout New York and many other cities across the United States. Though the world was in lockdown due to the coronavirus pandemic, people were drawn from their homes into the streets. Christopher and I made time to connect over the phone. I found myself anticipating the phone call in a way I had never anticipated a call with my longtime colleague and friend. While such violent acts against and upon Black bodies were not new in our country or our world, this was not something that Christopher and I had regularly brought into our many and varied conversations, directly. A position of privilege that I could take as a white woman, that is, to somehow, unconsciously, compartmentalize my work as a Jungian analyst, and psychoanalyst. To regard my friend and colleague in a way that did not explicitly consider our literal differences and the ways in which our contexts varied and how this would inevitably impact the way we work as analysts. Christopher, a Black man from Springfield, Massachusetts and, me, a white woman from Houston, Texas.

We shared a similar trajectory after we left our respective homes, which included postgraduate seminary training followed by doctoral studies at Union Theological Seminary (NYC), and a life of working in the not-for-profit sector in New York City before making the turn toward becoming Jungian analysts. But the lives we lived were filled with experiences and stories shaped by our own sets of racialized encounters of growing up in vastly different places within the United States from diverse perspectives, with dissimilar upbringings and surroundings. It became apparent to me, as I awaited our phone call, that the veil of silence was ripped wide open. We could not, not talk about this, anymore. I noted my own pulse rate, the heat rising in my face, my breath growing shallow. A complex was getting activated, is how we Jungians would describe it.

'How are you?', I asked Christopher when we first get on the call. 'Livid', he answered, slowly. Then silence followed. I noticed my breathing. I was suddenly paralyzed. What do I ask? What do I not ask? What do I say? How do I respond? Relate? Listen? Share? I was out for a walk in my neighborhood in northern Manhattan when we got on the call. A few minutes in, a rather violent and sudden thunderstorm broke, and our conversation was accompanied by the skies opening wide. An utter downpour ensued. I was now trudging through rivers of water rushing upon the greenway. Something was dissolving, internally, collectively, and between Christopher and me. Something that has continued to propel us forward, closer in our work together within our institute and within our friendship as I can no longer not see, and we can no longer not speak.

After Floyd's murder, many of us in our analytic community committed to meeting every other week to converse toward some understanding of how we, as analysts and people in the United States, respond to such evils that we find ourselves amidst and that we find within our own selves. This process group (about ten of us in total) continues to meet to discuss personal material, ways in which we find ourselves implicated within systemic injustice—our own biases and projections that arise within our work with patients, within our own lives outside of our offices, and in our own thinking and feeling.

About a year into our working together, Christopher's article was published and together the process group decided to facilitate a discussion on this article, as a follow up to his previous presentations to our community. This on-going process group helped to facilitate a discussion amongst the larger community of the JPA, during one of our colloquium weekends. After this discussion, Christopher approached me with the idea of this book, I was honored to collaborate.

I am indebted to Christopher for his candidness, friendship, love, thorough editorship, and dedication to this project, the one that we have coagulated here in this book and the one with which we are in partnership within our Jungian community. I am profoundly humbled by the work that the contributing authors, whom I am privileged to also call my friends, have put into each chapter. This is not light work. It is not easy work. It has required each of us, at various times, to address honestly and directly when we are caught or activated. Many of us have processed our work on these chapters in various ways, with one another, the content, and the process itself. Christopher and I have had to grapple with our own responses to how we read, hear, and remember differently at times, what activates each of us about the different writings and their renderings. We have worked to really listen and share with one another. I have been challenged, called-out and called-in by my friend and colleague. I have learned to see differently because of our working together. The project has been a work of healing, I believe, for our community of the JPA in New York City. We are eager to see how it will impact the Jungian community and the field of psychoanalysis at large as we urge our colleagues to cease the silence around the reality of systemic racism and how it pervades our field and our work in ways to which we remain unconscious.

While Jung's theory, in and of itself, is robust in its articulation of the other within, Jungian training programs (and psychoanalytic training programs, overall) lack a history of doing the concrete work of scouring our ways of working within the very theory by which we are so compelled and transformed. We have failed to ask: 'In what ways do we perpetuate sameness and exclude difference from our very offices, from our clinics, and from our training programs and paradigms?' In what ways are we complicit with systemic racism, in terms of how we teach and how we work? How are we *analysts* implicated by this lack?

The structure of this book

We open this volume with 'Time for Space at the Table'. Carter first published this work near the end of his psychoanalytic training, from the perspective of an African American of Native American ancestry (2021). He urges psychoanalytic training programs, mental health professions and medical professions to re-educate the collective society, to promote the discontinued implementation of race theory and the disuse of 'race' in our systems of categorizing and diagnosing, which he identifies as the cornerstone of the attitude of white supremacy, systematized racism, and many implicit biases that negatively impact our perceptions and understanding of human potentiality.

The second chapter, 'The Paradox of the Primitive and Jung's Relation to "Negroes"', is written by the prolific psychoanalytic writer Ann Ulanov, who also mentored both editors through our respective doctoral journeys. Ulanov explores Jung's paradoxical relation to the primitive layer of psyche and his relation to 'Negroes' whom he locates there. Jung finds negative and positive aspects of this primitive level of psyche that exists in all of us and forms a vital taproot of the unconscious. She draws implications for deepening the teaching of analysts in training.

Our third chapter, 'The Smoking Mirror', is written by Deborah Fausch, current president of the Jungian Psychoanalytic Association and a certified Jungian analyst in private practice in Mexico and New York City. Fausch explores the archetypal resonance of the color black, beginning with a short resume of the 'color complex' of the United States and its roots in English natural philosophy and history. She reveals a historical view of black that is connected to an archetypal base and contains innately opposing dynamics. She ends her chapter with an analytical challenge proffered as the question, 'Can this enriched idea of blackness help to heal the racial trauma of the United States and its black and white citizens?'

Sherry Salman, a founding member and the first president of the Jungian Psychoanalytic Association and a supervising and training analyst within our community, authors our fourth chapter, 'On Failings'. Her central question is, 'How will Jungian communities act in relation to our own dirt?' Salman discusses the *how* and *why* of, what she identifies as, Jung's failure to apply crucial aspects of his theory to himself as he encountered what was other within him, within other people, and within African traditions in Africa. She finds that such failures resulted in Jung's use of limiting, racially biased statements about black-skinned people. She argues that those culturally determined failures have mythic and archetypal components that may eventually induce mortification and mourning, when properly faced. Salman informs us that, if consciously held, those components may result in a reconstitution of a larger personality. The tension between regressive restoration of persona and corrective trickster dynamics is central to this argument. She argues it is left to the present and next generations to do what Jung did not—to more fully re-collect the projections that form in relating to other cultures. With urgency, we need to ritualize disruption and renewal, creating containers in which the dirt that the trickster throws in our faces may serve as compost for that which will nourish future generations.

In chapter 5, analytic author, Visiting Professor of Pastoral and Contextual Theology (University of the South), and Analyst-in-Training, Amy Bentley Lamborn offers 'From Ghost to Ancestor'. Lamborn writes on what she identifies as Jung's racial complex, viewing it as a ghost that has haunted generations of Jungians. She explores the transformation of this ghost into an ancestor who bequeaths a model of the transformation processes, disclosing his personal confrontations with the unconscious via *The Red Book* and *The Black Books*. As Jung learned to dwell with 'ghostly procession of the past', he exemplifies how an *anamnesis* of all that has been excluded/unlived may render a deeper healing of what Adrianne Harris (2012) and Helen Morgan (2021) call racism's *psychose blanche*. Lamborn asserts that the alchemical transmutation of archetypal whiteness amplifies the archetypal account of such an anamnesis, an *opus contra naturum*—the *opus* through which Jung's ghost is transformed into an ancestral spirit.

Chapter 6, 'The Whiteness Complex', is a contribution from another one of our analysts-in-training John Michael Hayes, who is also a practicing psychologist, psychoanalyst, and Episcopal priest in Maryland. Hayes offers Jung's presciently unique endowment to psychoanalytic theory, the complex theory, as a resource in deciphering systemic racism. Coming from his own personal experience, he finds *Whiteness* to be a cultural complex that blinds us and constellates unreflective attitudes and believes that affirm white superiority. He asserts that these attitudes and beliefs ignore contradictory evidence and disavows the horrific facts of history. Metacognitive awareness of the *whiteness complex* unfolds the possibility of transcending the complex's limitations, permitting us to see more actuality, and promotes fuller relationships.

Tiffany Houck, the current Director of Training at the Jungian Psychoanalytic Association, is the author of our seventh chapter, 'The Sunken Place'. Her chapter begins with Jordan Peele's portrayal of *the sunken place* from *Get Out* (2017) as an amplification of what she understands to be an archetypal root of the cultural complex, white supremacy. Using Carl G. Jung's paradigm, she critiques a dominant, unconscious phenomenon within analytic training and analytic practice which is resultant of that which Resmaa Menakem (2017) describes as *dirty pain*—the pain of avoidance, blame, and denial. She finds that Peele's film, and the Black Horror genre (Bellot 2021) in general, can be understood as a modern-day mythology that amplifies an unconsciously known, but consciously not-thought-about experience of systemic racism in America that moves the audience closer to feeling the pain and grief of white body supremacy trauma. This chapter concludes with a look at Michael Rothberg's (2019) notion of the implicated subject offering a roadmap for how a majority-white Jungian analytic learning community might begin to take up the difficult work of anti-racism.

Our eighth and final chapter, 'Reparative Transgression', is written by Sarah J. Braun, a psychiatrist and Jungian analyst in Philadelphia. She is also an analyst member of the Jungian Psychoanalytic Association (New York). Braun draws upon the personal significance of the process that psychoanalytic communities engaged in during the 1990s to confront anti-Semitism. She addresses current attempts to face destructive effects of racism in Jung's writings and in the teaching and practices of analytical psychology. Reflecting on how, as a member of a training community, she has both engaged and been paralyzed by the necessity to reckon this taboo reality. Braun highlights transgression's paradoxical nature, as is evident in the individuation process—transgression plays a parallel role in causing harm and in making reparation. She shares features of the Jewish Holiday of Passover in depicting psychological processes that can shift individuals and groups from paralysis into engagement. Braun informs us that there is an ethical imperative for psychoanalysts and training communities to engage in voluntarily intentional processes of self-examination toward reparation, contributing to greater wholeness in the collective.

In many ways, race is the cornerstone to an impersonal system that affects people on a very personal level. The contributions within this work weave into a tapestry of lived experiences. *Jungian Reflections on Systemic Racism* takes-up Jung's theories of the complex, individuation, primitivity, dissociation, projection, and recollection to decipher and interpret unconscious racial bias and racism within Jung's writings, within psychoanalytic training programs, and within psychoanalytic practices.

Race has many associations. In some ways, the concept beckons images of heritage and pride. In other ways, it is a complicated barrier with no clear point of entry. We ask that readers approach this work in the spirit of curiosity, concern and with such compassion that one is patient with oneself, but does not deflect the opportunity to approach this work with one eye looking outward while the other eye reflects inwardly upon the reader's personal history and processes in response to the image, *race*.

References

Bellot, G. (2021). 'How Black Horror Became America's Most Powerful Cinematic Genre', *The New York Times Style Magazine*. https://www.nytimes.com/2021/11/10/t-magazine/black-horror-films-get-out.html

Brewster, F. (2017). *African Americans and Jungian Psychology: Leaving the Shadows.* Abingdon: Routledge.

Carter, C. J. (2021). 'Time for Space at the Table: An African-American/Native-American Analyst-in-training's First-hand Reflections. A Call for the IAAP to Publicly Denounce (But Not Erase) the White Supremacist Writings of C.G. Jung'. *Journal of Analytical Psychology*, 66, I, 70–92.

Dalal, F. (1988). 'Jung: A Racist'. *British Journal of Psychotherapy*, 4, 263–279.

Harris, A. (2012). 'The House of Difference, or White Silence'. *Studies in Gender and Sexuality*, 13, 197–216.

Jung, C. G. (2009). *The Red Book. Liber Novus, A Reader's Edition*, ed. S. Shamdasani. New York & London: W.W. Norton.

Menakem, R. (2017). *My Grandmother's Hands: Racialized Trauma and the Pathway to Mending Our Hearts and Bodies.* Las Vegas, NV: Central Recovery Press.

Morgan, H. (2021). *The Work of Whiteness: A Psychoanalytic Perspective.* London and New York: Routledge.

'Open Letter from a Group of Jungians on the Question of Jung's Writings on and Theories about "Africans"'. (2018). *British Journal of Psychotherapy*, 34, 4, 673–678.

Peale, J. (2017). *Get Out.* Universal Pictures.

Rothberg, M. (2019). *The Implicated Subject: Beyond Victims and Perpetrators.* Stanford: Stanford University Press.

Ulanov, Ann Belford. (2014). *Knots and their Untying: Essays on Psychological Dilemmas.* New Orleans: Spring Journal Books.

Chapter 1

Time for Space at the Table

An African American-Native American psychoanalyst's first-hand reflections. A call for the IAAP to publicly denounce (but not erase) the White supremacist writings of C.G. Jung[1]

Christopher Jerome Carter

The alchemist's formula 'Their gold is not our gold' holds true; but this is not to say their dross is not our dross. I ask the reader to hold the attitude Jung presented in seeking the foundation stone of the building: 'I would like to kick the garbage away from me, if the golden seed were not in the vile heart of the misshapen form' (Jung 2009, 139, p. 424. 164/165).

A man of his time?

Between 2016 and 2019 (my first three years of classes as an analyst-in-training), I and a colleague (a woman of color) had shared relatively open-minded responses to Jung's written misperceptions of non-Europeans as 'primitives'. Jung specifically targets the Negro and the Red man as primitive, with a particular tone of distain for the Negro. All of my questions and feedback regarding Jung's mercurial applications of the term primitive were speedily deflected with the ever lackluster, 'Jung was a man of his time'. The offence adheres. All are deeply influenced by time. There remains a wide spectrum of attitudes and choices.

Perhaps to supplement the hollow excuse, (white) instructors would then boast that Jung's passion for mythology and psychoanalytic exploration motivated his travels and his reported immersions in foreign cultures, more fully witnessing the *Unus Mundus*. There seems to be some comfort in justifying and redirecting Jung's offences. It is as though Jung illustrated that the celebration of individuality forfeits social responsibility. Complaints against Jung's offensiveness get into discussions about projection and projective-identification. Many Jungians secure the provisional life by shielding their alliances and denying any objective role they may play in external (ized) torment. Ironically, Jung writes, 'As long as it is a provisional life, your unconscious will be in a state of continuous irritation against you' (Jung 1931, p. 194).

In her essay, 'Jung on the Provisional Life' (2014), Sue Mehrtens provides a pertinent description of Jung's hypothesis of the provisional life. 'Provisional life' denotes 'the Modern European disease of the merely imaginary life' (Jung 30 Aug. 1931, 'Letter to Count Hermann Keyserling'),[2] a life lacking investment

DOI: 10.4324/9781003311447-2

in the hard news of external reality. After enduring a heart attack and experiencing an apocalyptic vision near 1944, Jung wrote, "I no longer attempt to put across my own opinion, but surrendered myself to the current of my thoughts'. Reportedly, he also developed:

> An affirmation of things as they are: an unconditional 'yes' to that which is, without subjective protests — acceptance of the conditions of existence as I see them and understand them, acceptance of my own nature, as I happen to be …. It was only after the illness that I understood how important it is to affirm one's own destiny. In this way we forge an ego that does not break down when incomprehensible things happen; an ego that endures, that endures the truth, and that is capable of coping with the world and with fate.
>
> (Jung 1961/1989, p. 297)

The above is exemplary of the senex's wise regard for provisional living. But balance is warranted. The 'race' lie is an impairment to the great majority of Black and Brown folks. We witness racist dynamics reverberating towards annihilating non-white individuality, gaslighting non-Whites into accepting sub-standards of living and dying. My mind, body, soul, and spirit reject the notion of an unconditional 'yes' to things as they are. Love and compassion tolerate conditions. Unfortunately, analysts who would turn a blind eye to the impact of bigotry might experience my process of differentiating the personal from the collective and of aligning more with my unique individuality (individuation) as threatening — a menace to the provisional life.

Denying the influence of Jung's White supremacist writings fosters Social Darwinism, as though to justify racism and inequity. Darwin's theory was often misapplied to human cultures and ethnicities, as though to exemplify different species within humanity, with *pure*, White Europeans as The Prize of Creation. I find no pleasure in identifying another as a White supremacist, especially when the subject has not publicly self-identified as such and I have never interacted with them. Contrary to being talion, mapping the attitudes and influences of a very powerful man grants the IAAP opportunities for greater practical and theoretical balance: "Racial identifications that maintain whiteness as a construct privileged over otherness are an obstacle to conducting analytic work' (Powell 2018, p. 1021). Such an obstacle puts us in a position of preaching what we cannot put into practice, 'for we do not hold the opposites and hear the tension, consciously, thus inhabiting a space between. We sever instead' (Ulanov 2014, p. 129).

In defining White supremacy and White supremacism, an appropriately inclusive definition is offered by legal scholar Francis Lee Ansley:

> By "white supremacy" I do not mean to allude only to the self-conscious racism of white supremacist hate groups. I refer instead to a political,

economic and cultural system in which whites overwhelmingly control power and material resources, conscious and unconscious ideas of white superiority and entitlement are widespread, and relations of white dominance and non-white subordination are daily reenacted across a broad array of institutions and social settings.

(Ansley 1989, pp. 933–34)

One may find the term 'white supremacist' to be jarring and affect-laden. To the open bigot, the term evokes a sense of pride. The term usually refers to those who subscribe to racist beliefs and who revel in humiliating and oppressing others to advance 'white power'. Participation in the propaganda and activities of an established group is not a prerequisite for an attitude of white supremacy.

Alas, many of Jung's writings are soiled with pejorative declarations that add nothing to analytic theory, but belittle, demean and propagandize against non-Europeans, with a special intolerance toward African Americans. Jung prioritized *Whiteness* as that which needed to be shielded from contamination. Jung's expressed attitude towards people of color was often consonant with white supremacy.

This matter is crucial because Jung was, and remains, powerfully authoritative. Those who revere Jung as a sage may wonder, 'Who am I to question someone who probed the psychic depths and articulated them with such *compos mentis*?' Those who fully align with Jung (as opposed to those who eat the meat and spit out the bones) may identify with his supremacist attitude. This may be ego-dystonic, but:

> The attitude or disposition, then, can thrust itself on consciousness from outside or from inside, like an affect, and can therefore be expressed by the same figures of speech. An attitude seems, at first glance, to be something very much more complicated than an affect. On closer inspection, however, we find that this is not so, because most attitudes are based, consciously or unconsciously, on some kind of maxim, which often has the character of a proverb. In some attitudes one can immediately detect the underlying maxim and even discover where it was picked up. Often the attitude is distinguished only by a single word, which as a rule stands for an ideal. Not infrequently, the quintessence of an attitude is neither a maxim nor an ideal but a personality who is revered and emulated.
>
> (Jung 1926, para. 631)

In 'The Complications of American Psychology', originally titled, 'Your Negroid and Indian Behavior', Jung states:

> Racial infection is a most serious mental and moral problem where the primitive outnumbers the white man. America has this problem only in a relative degree, because the whites far outnumber the coloured. Apparently,

he can assimilate the primitive influence with little risk to himself. What would happen if there were a considerable increase in the coloured population is another matter.

(Jung 1930, para. 966)

As analytic theory evolved, an attitudinal shift in Jung was exemplified in a less deprecatory application of 'primitive'. Perhaps this reveals tension between his soul and a racist alignment: 'somewhere you are the same as the Negro or the Chinese or whoever you live with, you are all just human beings' (Jung 1935, para. 93). But Jung whitewashes the collective psyche's universality, promoting white supremacy: 'It matters to a certain extent, sure enough—he probably has a whole historical layer less than you. The different strata of the mind correspond to the history of the races' (ibid.).

It is hard to trust that Jung remained oblivious to the heroism in Black narratives, having studied the Negro. Did Jung overlook Frederick Douglass, who was born into enslavement (1817; Tuckahoe, MD), escaping when he was nearly 21 years old? Douglass's well-circulated words resonated throughout Europe. Jung was near 19 years old when Douglass said:

We have amongst us, those who have taken the first prizes as scholars; those who have won distinction for courage and skill on the battlefield; those who have taken rank as lawyers, doctors and ministers of the gospel; those who shine among men in every useful calling; and yet we are called 'a problem ... a disturbing force, threatening destruction to the holiest and best interests of society.

(Douglass 1984, p. 36)

Jung acknowledges neither the social contributions nor the scientific advancements of Africans and American descendants of Africans. In 'Jung in the African diaspora', Vaughan (2019) notes that Jung travelled to the United States several times between 1909 and 1937 but appeared ignorant of the American legal system's impact on African American society and culture. Jung turned a blind eye to the Harlem Renaissance 'and the inherent contradictions and challenges it would have posed for his thinking and writing about African Americans and others in the African diaspora ... . Perhaps he chose not to see' (Vaughan 2019, pp. 334, 336).

Jung oversteps in suggesting that the secretive rites of the Ku Klux Klan are 'analogous to any primitive mystery religion', and maybe as effective as shamanism.

Secret societies of every description abound all over the county from the Ku Klux Klan to the Knights of Columbus, and their rites are analogous to any primitive mystery religion. America has resuscitated the ghosts of Spiritualism, of which she is the original home, and cures diseases by

Christian Science, which has more to do with the shaman's mental healing than with any recognizable kind of science. Moreover, it is proving to be pretty effective, just as were the cures of the shaman.

(Jung 1930, para. 977)

'Moreover it is proving to be pretty effective, just as were the cures of the shaman' refers directly to Christian Science. The overall question of this chapter is how 'roughness, brutality and primitivity', which Jung identified as originating in the *Negro* and the *Red Man*, has 'infected' white Americans. It is excruciating to witness whites side-track this factor in our discussions. It has been as though white instructors have preconsciously attempted to gas-light me into crediting Jung's comparison by accepting the overall assault. As Fields and Fields report, 'Disguised as race, racism becomes something Afro-Americans are, rather than something racists do. Racists and apologist have long availed themselves of the deception' (2012/2014, pp. 96–97).

Contending that primal infections fester in American initiations, secret societies and Spiritualism, Jung turns a blind eye to the uncompromisingly bigoted and murderous purview of the KKK. Discussing that organization without centralizing its collective attitude and mission is an offence that does not soften with time. Even more hostile is the misinformed notion that the KKK's separatist rites, often ripe with homicidal ideation (at best), were ever analogous to the ancestor-honoring, community-building, outcast-redeeming rites of Negroes and Native Americans. I have debated this error with training instructors. Remember: 'Not infrequently, the quintessence of an attitude is ... a personality who is revered and emulated' (Jung 1926, para. 631).

Through the fallacy of bio-racism, biases are reified as though they are aligned with nature. It may be beneficial to rework Jung's hypotheses re-garding nature's impact on the individual psyche and regarding the impact of cultural cross-pollination on the development of the collective psyche (including *participation mystique*).

Jung's findings on the personal psyche, the collective psyche, and the risks of unhealthy inflation are intriguing. Healthy inflation occurs as the personal is differentiated from the collective. The subject then comes to realize the great paradox of wealth-emptiness that reverberates within the depths. As internal resources expand, the individual is daringly differenti-ated from the herd.

By raising the personal unconscious to consciousness, the analysis makes the subject aware of things which he is generally aware of in others, but never in himself. This discovery makes him less individually unique, and more collective ... . The lifting of personal repressions at first brings purely personal contents into consciousness; but attached to them are the collective elements of the unconscious, the ever-present instincts, qualities, and ideas (images) as well as all those 'statistical' quotas of average virtue and average vice which we recognize when we say, 'Everyone has in him something of the criminal, the genius, and the saint' ... . A sense of solidarity with the world is gradually built up, which is felt by many natures as something very positive and in certain cases actually is the deciding factor in the treatment of neurosis.

(Jung 1928, para. 236)

Jung depicts the fruits of efficacious analysis exquisitely, balancing the personal and the collective. Analytic theory proposes that binaries (*coincidentia oppositorum*) arise within the psyche to stoke tensions that promote an 'as though' new path and a new attitude. A promotional tension of correspondences is virtually absent from Jung's 'race' discourse.

There are Mercurial incongruities in Jung's cultural contamination conjecture, particularly in terms of 'race'. The collective psyche pertains to portions of every psyche that are innately rooted, universally impersonal and suprapersonal. Those who incorporate material of the collective psyche as though it were *on a par* with personally acquired experiences suffer an unhealthy personality inflation. This happens because the collective psyche, the basis of every personality, houses *les parties inférieures* of psychic functioning. When at the helm, *les parties inférieures* result either in the 'stifling of self-confidence or else in an unconscious heightening of the ego's importance to the point of a pathological will to power'. A healthy personality requires 'strict differentiation from the collective psyche ... since partial or blurred differentiation leads to an immediate melting away of the individual in the collective'. Such a bleeding of the collective psyche over the domains of the personal psyche leads to a feeling of universal validity 'which completely ignores all differences in the personal psyche of his fellows' (Jung 1928, para. 235). Here is the point of incongruity:

A collective attitude naturally presupposes this same collective psyche in others. But that means a ruthless disregard not only of individual differences but also of differences of a more general kind within the collective psyche itself, as for example differences of races ... . The element of differentiation is the individual.

(Jung 1928, para. 240)

The collective psyche, when superimposed on the personal psyche and regarded as ontogenetically developed, leads to an attitude that presupposes the same collective psyche in others. He writes this in the same document in which he declares that the collective psyche is universal and in every individual's psyche. Perhaps it would have been more clarifying to write, 'A collective attitude naturally presupposes this same collective attitude in others?' Such a distinction would avoid equating one's awareness of the collective psyche with the detrimental attitude. With what rationale does Jung subdivide the universal collective psyche into the 'more general kind of differences in the collective psyche', and how is 'race' to be regarded? How is race segregated in the collective psyche when 'All the highest achievements of virtue, as well as the blackest villainies, are individual' (ibid., para. 240, pp. 152–53)?

The offence of racism permeates much of Jung's work. This attitude leaves the other-than-White analyst-in-training with the burden of parallel processing the bigotry they are instructed to metabolize in Jung and the racist micro-aggressions of their training program. Unaddressed, this matter is a whitewash that promotes torment. Borrowing Helen Morgan's citation of the definition of 'whitewash' from *The Chamber's Dictionary*:

> 'to cover with whitewash; to give a fair appearance to; to take steps to clear the stain from (a reputation), cover up (an official misdemeanor) or rehabilitate (a person) in the public eye; to beat (an opponent) so decisively in a game that he or she fails to score at all.'
>
> (Morgan 2004, p. 217)

The last meaning is particularly acerbic. It reflects the unholy glow of racism, concentrated in standardized race doctrine. I am not offering an in-depth etymology of race, but the concept may have emerged between 1730 and 1790 to serve the colonial enterprises of European powers, classifying groups based on regional origin, skin colour and physical differences (Kennedy 2013, p. xiii). Regarding the concept of race in psychology, Graham Richards asserts:

> It indeed arose in relation to the 'transfactual' reality of human physical diversity but it now appears as if there was never any 'transfactual' phenomenon to which the term itself referred. For Psychology ... we are concerned with the ineluctably moral question of the psychological nature of the 'race' concept as a psychological phenomenon in its own right. My earlier distinction between 'racialism' and 'racism' may thus be recouched as one between 'necessary' and 'contingent' racism. 'Necessary' racism (my 'racialism') occurs because, given Psychology's reflexive nature, psychologists who are members of culturally and psychologically racist communities will necessarily share that community's psychological character in some degree ... . Even the most self-consciously 'anti-racist' people may appear retrospectively racist in this sense.
>
> (Richards 1997, pp. xiii–xiv)

The whitewash's efficacy is in the universalization of the 'transfactual' factor (race). Richards does not address Jung, but he writes extensively on psychology's role in promoting 'scientific racism'. Race is an ideology originally designed to justify (as though scientifically) the pillaging, raping and enslavement of people of color for the overall domination and prosperity of Whites. The notion of 'race' is central to White supremacy. The whitewashing and the gaslighting remain efficacious because it is easy to mistake actual factors of 'racism' (colorism) for the lie, 'race'. According to historians Karen E. Fields and Barbara J. Fields,

'Race' too often recommends itself as a guiltless word, a neutral term for an empirical fact. It is not. Race appears to be a neutral description of reality because of the race-racism evasion, through which immoral acts of discrimination disappear, and then reappear camouflaged as the victim's alleged difference.

(Fields & Fields 2012/2014, p. 95)

Depth psychology has largely eliminated Africanist myths from view. How might the myths and narratives of survivors and descendants of the African diaspora inform the process of individuation and the development of the collective psyche? Jungian psychology has made little space for such explorations. As Fanny Brewster writes:

Jungian psychology as it is practiced has a profound attachment to considerations of our ancestors and how they influence us in contemporary life ... . It might seem insignificant to think about the consciousness of how we perceive our skin but in the narrative of racial relations and racism in the American collective, skin as culture has been and continues to be vitally important ... . In considering the 'underneath' of the body and our desire to preserve it or release it through death, there are cultural considerations that are dependent upon traditional spiritual and philosophical beliefs.

(Brewster 2019, pp. 308–09)

There is something insidious about Jung's writings on Blacks and their spirituality in the absence of Africanist myths. His opus discredits our capacity to introspect and to mentalize. Jung's opus mocks the Africanist's culture(s) and spirituality with a tone that aligns with Uncle Remus stories – denigrating folklore that is fueled by cultural incompetency. Such a perspective lacks scientific value and only serves as a passive aggressive allegory in support of a scruffily structured theoretical point.

For instance, that famous story: A nigger is sick and naturally he asks himself what that comes from; it is perfectly unnatural to be sick, therefore it must have been caused by witchcraft, perhaps the tin fetish he is carrying round his neck has lost its magical efficiency, or he has given offence to some unknown ghost or demon, or to a sorcerer of a foreign tribe. At first, he may not be able to remember the magical reason for his disease, but it certainly has a magical reason for not even death is natural to a nigger, it is always caused by witchcraft.

(Jung 1931, p. 211)

Here, as remains true in Jung's 'time', we are actually talking about space ... space away from any threat to the white psyche. An insular nationalist who dreaded *blackness*, it appears that Jung made no space for respectful engagement.

Long before Jung was established as an authority, Douglass was vocal about such distorted imagery that whites attached onto blackness:

> When a black man's language is quoted, in order to belittle and degrade him, his ideas are put into the most grotesque and unreadable English, while the utterances of negro scholars and authors are ignored. A hundred white men will attend a concert of white negro minstrels with faces blackened with burnt cork, to one who will attend a lecture by an intelligent negro.
>
> (Douglass 1894, p. 19)

It is good to differentiate and celebrate colors, ethnicities, cultures and traditions. But the very concept of race is racist. Jung and other white supremacists dreaded the risk of a hypothetical psychic contamination that might occur through the intermingling of cultures and ethnicities. Such dreadful ideas persist today. This is unfortunate, misguided and is of no value to analytic theory, unless the focus is on the psychology of the bigot.

We can all lay claim to unconscious biases. One way of getting hold of one's biases is to become increasingly cognizant of the gravity of (mis) perceptions, the true impact of one's attitude in motivating harmful behaviors (i.e., espousing racist propaganda). In transforming unconscious bias into cognitive bias, one may experience an increase in relationality with those slippery, shadowy aspects of the self that are readily projected, thereby introjecting the abject that may contain metaphorical gold, aligning one to a path towards greater wholeness.

It is unproductive to assert that Jung was unconsciously biased about his racist views. He was quite cognizant of his biases and repeatedly stood behind them in his writings [full-stop]. The question of unconscious bias is more relevant to Jungian analysts and analysts in training: if we embrace the totality of C. G. Jung's thought in an undifferentiated way, might we see black as inferior? Might we perpetuate such antiquated biases in analytic theory and practice?

Exemplified space for the respectful engagement of Jung's white supremacist views

For whatever ulterior motives he may have had, Dalal (1988) clearly spells-out Jung's repeated attacks on people of African descent, and quite often enough towards Blacks. To paraphrase Dalal, Jung tends to:

i   equate Blacks with primitive
ii equate Black consciousness with the white unconscious
iii equate the Black adult with the white child

I might disagree with Dalal if he is implying that Jung's biases permeate the core of either Jungian theory or practice. Yet, clearly racist writings and statements are interwoven in Jung's discussion of the collective unconscious and individuation. Race biology is a pseudoscience that was discredited in the second half of the 20th century (United Nations Educational, Scientific and Cultural Organization 1950). It only detracts from analytic theory. Nevertheless, in 1954 Jung approved a transcript that would eventually be published two months after his death. The transcript was of a discussion with The Guild of Pastoral Psychology. It includes, 'I have been led by dreams, like any primitive. I am, ashamed to say so, but I am as primitive as any nigger*, because I do not know' (Jung 1939, para. 674). The offence* is justified in footnote 11: 'This offensive term was not invariably derogatory in earlier British and Continental usage, and definitely not in this case'. Talk about *false truths*! One of many racist comments, that line of thinking aligns with a more violent comment Jung made in a 1932 seminar (approximately 70 years after the Emancipation Proclamation). It is an unapologetic comment without an asterisk:

> Certain people deserve that you shall not be kind. You are indulging your own autoerotic pleasure, warming yourself by the thought of your wonderful kindness, but you are wronging those people, you are leading them more into error. So, you need a certain amount of cruelty. Those Negroes are murderous devils, who might kill other people as well as yourself, so why should they be free? They had far better be chained.
>
> (Jung 1932, p. 681)

Jung maintained this attitude some 23 years after the Freud–Jung lectures at the 1909 Clark University conference. Jung stood no more than seven bodies in front of America's first African American psychiatrist, Solomon Carter Fuller (1872–1953) in a group photo for the event coordinated by the university's president, G. Stanley Hall. The only person of color to attend those lectures, 'Fuller was Hall's personal physician and perhaps his analyst, and there was evidence that Fuller corresponded with Freud' (Powell 2018, p. 1026). Fuller, then a pioneer in the study of Alzheimer's disease, was also a speaker at the conference (Terry 2008).

Some 36 years before Jung's Visions seminars, Douglass lectured on the injustices hurled upon Blacks and the complaint that Blacks were America's societal problem. In doing so, he provided greater perspective on human development through reflecting upon Black progress. Douglass rendered a first-person testimony that could have illuminated analytic theory, had Jung been unfettered to White supremacism. The complaint was called the Negro problem ... the dread that emancipated Black and Brown people would cause the decline of American society. Douglass displays a degree of acuity in matters concerning the psychological development of the collective:

> I reject the charge brought against the negro as a class, because all through the late war, while the slave masters of the South were absent from their homes ... with the vile purpose of perpetuating the enslavement of the negro, their wives, their daughters, their sisters and their mothers were left in the absolute custody of these same negroes ... when the negro had every opportunity to commit the abominable crime now alleged against him, there was never a single instance of such crime reported or charged against him ... in the whole South ... Then, again on general principles, I do not believe the charge because it implies an improbable, if not an impossible change in mental and moral character and composition of the negro. It implies a change wholly inconsistent with well-known facts of human nature. It is a contradiction to well-known human experience. History does not present an example of such a transformation in the character of any class of men ... . Decline in the moral character of a people is not sudden, but gradual. The downward steps are marked at first by degrees and by increasing momentum from bad to worse ... and I contend that the negroes of the South have not had time to experience this great change and reach this lower depth of infamy. On the contrary, in point of fact, they have been and still are, improving and ascending to higher levels of moral and social worth.
>
> (Douglass 1894, p. 11)

Could there be an unaddressed attitude within the field of psychoanalysis that makes BIPOC (Black, Indigenous and People of Color) folk feel as though we are imposters as we attempt to sit at the table for an equitable education towards personal development and the promotion of a healthier society (albeit via the individual)? I have visited other training institutes. I venture to say I am not alone. No doubt, I belong at the table. But something has been off. There is history behind it. Basking in misaligned god-likeness, white supremacists systematically dehumanized enslaved Africans to root inferiority within the personalities or Black and Brown people, for all eternity. Clinical psychologist Na'im Akbar (1984) identifies a sense of inferiority as one of the most destructive characteristics from slavery. He finds that this characteristic girds the Eurocentric psychological tradition, with psychologists utilizing this characteristic more than anyone else as 'an explanation for nearly every aspect of African-American behavior'. In 1903, W. E. B. Du Bois (1868–1963) wrote:

> And above all, we daily hear that an education that encourages aspiration, that sets the loftiest of ideals and seeks as an end culture and character,

rather than bread-winning, is the privilege of white men and the danger and delusion of black.

(Du Bois 1903/1989, pp. 78–79)

The systematic dehumanization of Blacks is on display in Jung's writings, mired in bigotry. In 1931:

> The primitive, for instance, ordinarily has no psychology; there are no such figures or occurrences because there is no space, no chance for it. The very primitive man is still identical with the collective unconscious, he is just a piece of the world, a part of visible nature, and values himself as one among the other animals.

(Jung 1931, p. 211)

Akbar quotes the American historian, author, journalist and founder of the Association for the Study of African American Life and History, Carter G. Woodson (1875–1950):

> To handicap a student for life by teaching him that his black face is a curse and that his struggle to change his conditions is hopeless, is the worst kind of lynching. It kills one's aspirations and dooms him to vagabondage and crime.

(Akbar 1984, p. 21)

We must verbalize, document and demonstrate that we embrace much of Jung's analytic theory but we do not embrace the continued dehumanization of BIPOC people. Individuation is contingent upon neither color, ethnicity, gender, sexuality, nationality, nor socio-economic factors. In differentiating our perspectives from Jung's, we utilize a wider lens to stimulate insight.

The benefits of opening dialogue on Jung and race in analytic training

Having had a full day of discussion about Jung and 'race' with the Jungian Psychoanalytic Association (14 July 2019), I do feel like I actually have a place at the table. No longer an imposter, I neither dread being perceived as 'going White' nor being assigned Jung's 'White complex in Negroes' as a hindrance to self-expression and greater individuation. There is room for confrontation when it makes an opening for the third. Via the analytic approach, there is room for all of my relations, our histories, our narratives, our myths, our songs, our prospects. All of Us.

In my analytic training, I am no longer preoccupied with the burden of Jung's prejudices. I cannot identify as a *Jungian* analyst-in-training; but as a candidate training-in-Jungian psychoanalysis. This is not a play on words.

I align with the theory more than the person, pondering how I might further integrate that shadow, that internal White supremacist, that nationalist, that colonizer. I cannot feel so aligned with one who never reconciled to me. I sense that Jung was a bit of an Archie Bunker.[3] But Archie taught us to lift up our differences in the light of day. The image of Archie beckons forth the intellect, to confront and process biases and fears. Perhaps what is being constellated is that conflict between *the spirit of the times* and *the spirit of the depths* that Jung identifies in *Liber Primus*? I am in Jungian training because the theory has efficacy and belongs to us all.

Following my training institutes' 'Jung & Race' panel discussion, I have observed that some course instructors who previously relied upon the standard 'Jung was a man of his time' are now increasingly engaging in ways that facilitate creative tensions toward healthier, fuller, and more inclusive dialogue. We appreciate the fact that heat is intrinsic to the topic, 'race'. We can disagree without disagreeable attitudes. We disclose our thoughts of how that which Jung disregarded might or might not inform analysis and analytic theory.

Time for the IAAP to make space for Black, Brown and First Nations People?

Should we refuse to acknowledge Jung's limitations, will it be out of the preconscious dread of parricide? Do we worry that the deconstruction of 'race' will result in the decline of analytical psychology (i.e. matricide)? Jung has informed us of the value of holding the tension of the opposites. We must see the other before a path toward the new can surface. There is a growing outcry against Jung's needlessly offensive writings. There is an unexplored tension in the tones of bigotry and misogyny that reverberate in writings that are uniquely formulated to promote wholeness. Does this tension reverberate in the symphonies of intolerance conducted by current world leaders, in real time–space?

On 2 February 2020, Ahmaud Arbury (25), an African-American and former high school football standout, was hunted and shot dead by Whites during a short jog in Satilla Shores, GA. His killers, arrested months later, filmed the assassination. The video captures a killer standing over Mr Arbury's body while hurling a violent racial slur (Fausset 2020).

On 1 March 2020, as the United States of America debated the actions that led to Arbury's death, New York State Governor Andrew Cuomo (2020) announced that New York State had identified its first case of COVID-19. As infection rates climbed dramatically on the West and East Coasts of the United States, Americans clutched to the refrain, 'We're all in this together', expressing solidarity and promoting prophylaxis.

Pandemics expose humanity's ephemerality. All of humanity, when unvarnished with privilege and excesses, is virtually on equal footing. I wondered if the pandemic would move a largely sequestered country to survey the connection between negative attitudes towards 'other' and nefarious behaviors. Yet, many leaders in the United States, Europe and other countries utilize confusion about the pandemic to further 'anti-immigrant, White supremacist, ultra-nationalist, anti-Semitic, and xenophobic conspiracy theories' (Human Rights Watch 2020). Donald Trump mirthfully mis-identifies COVID-19 as 'the Chinese virus'. It is as though equality threatens the bigot, so he gaslights the 'other' through terror and belittlement. This tsunami of 'hate and xeno-phobia, scapegoating and scare-mongering' (ibid.) expresses the racist pertur-bation – the contamination of 'White'.

On 13 March 2020, the African American emergency medical technician Breonna Taylor (26) was shot at least eight times in her apartment by White police officers reportedly executing a search warrant that did not require them to announce themselves before entry. Ms Taylor was without medical attention for more than 20 minutes, perhaps because medical personnel were occupied with aiding others struggling for breath due to COVID-19 (Duvall & Costello 2020). The official incident report stated that Ms Taylor had no injuries. Officers also denied forceful entry. As of 17 September 2020, the officers involved had not been charged (Oppel et al. 2020).

By 20 March 2020, Gov. Cuomo issued the 100% closure of non-essential businesses state-wide, effective Sunday, 22 March at 8 p.m. (Eastern Standard Time). Essential services included groceries, delivery services and healthcare. We celebrate the courageous stamina of essential workers, many being persons of color who risk their safety to sustain the collective. Higher percentages of Black and Brown folk were getting infected with COVID-19, partially because they conducted the humble work that is now deemed 'es-sential'. There was a mercurial air of equality in America. Perhaps justice for Arbury and Taylor would prevail! After all, 'We're all in this together'.

Bigotry reared its ugly head in broad daylight on 25 May. After a Minneapolis grocery store complained of receiving a counterfeit twenty-dollar bill, four White police officers responded and detained 46-year-old African American George Floyd, an unarmed hip hop artist and a mentor in his religious community. Handcuffed from behind, he was placed onto a street with Officer Derek Chauvin consistently kneeling on Mr Floyd's neck for 8 minutes and 15 seconds. Two other officers pinned his legs and back. Witnesses recorded the event, pleading that the officers were being too aggressive. A fourth officer kept witnesses back from Chauvin. The video captured Mr Floyd begging for relief, complaining, 'I can't breathe', and 'You're killing me!' As Floyd cried for his life, the video revealed Chauvin's appallingly apathetic face as he performed the lynching-by-knee. *The New York Times* investigated the full recording and found that Chauvin did not remove his knee even after Mr Floyd lost consciousness, continuing the lynching for a full minute and 20 seconds after paramedics arrived (Hill et al. 2020). The day after Mr Floyd's death, the Police Department fired all four of the officers involved in the episode. All four face charges for killing

Mr. Floyd. This graphic exhibition of savage bigotry nullified the slogan, 'We are all in this together'. White supremacism rouses in a silent majority until it detonates, as though 'heroically' exterminating blackness.

It was not until June that I realized White analysts could 'detach' from the trifecta of emotionally destabilizing factors: racism, COVID-19, and financial instability that has left record numbers of people with unemployment, food instability, and healthcare fears. Matters are far worse on many First Nations reservations that still lack running water and access to adequate health services. All but one of my current analysands have shared difficult dreams either pertaining to racism, to COVID-19, or to matters related to financial instability. Some analysts report that the topic of racism has never entered their practice, ever. Perhaps the analyst's attitude gaslights the matter from approachability, silencing the analysand.

My American training institute continues the dialogue on Jung and 'race' that began in July 2019. Many analysts express value in educating themselves on how implicit biases arise in analytic practice and influence analytic theory. Like most paradigms of psychology, analysis has a role in systemic racism. The IAAP can elect to take a role in the de-institutionalization of racism (deconstructing race), publicly demonstrating the value of holding the tensions between the personal and the collective, promoting the wellness of both, on a global scale.

We do not want to have our profession misidentified with the darkenss of bigotry; but there is no illumination in turning a blind eye. We experience the validity of analytic theory, inclusive of multiplicities and paradoxes. Jung demonstrated a lot of growth, although not without complications, in his understanding of 'primitive', and in his writings on Wotan (reflecting upon Nazi Germany). Neither he nor I could expect to embody the totality of the self. It is an ongoing journey.

I perceived a fear of contamination in one of the presentations during JPA's 2019 Winter Colloquium.[4] I felt compelled to tease it out during the question and answer period following the presentation. The presenter irradiated a sense of displacement experienced by landowners and those in power whose communities become infiltrated by foreign cultures, dramatically impacting their environments and ways of being. His presentation was thought-provoking. Professing to know little about psychoanalysis, the presenter displayed a type of kinship with Jung in his erudite approach to his work. This approach is highly prized in academia, and we accept a degree of arrogance (god-likeness) as characteristic of the learned. It is an arrogance that seems to prize differentiation but somehow misses the value of inclusion.

Jung is not alone. All fall short. All have biases, many of which remain secretive. In his time, Jung took internal explorations into new depths. In denying his superficial, publicly exposed weaknesses – misbeliefs that inadvertently promote current global pushes toward the restriction, the negation, and even the obliteration of 'Other' – we align with Jung's errors and bypass opportunities for greater social transformation. There is no "person of color" in the JPA who is not negatively affected by Jung's perceptions on race. It is time to look the error (white supremacy) in the eye, comprehending Jung's biases, unmasking ways in which white supremacist thought may be infused in analytic theory. This task begins with the deconstruction of 'race' (acknowledging that 'racists' and 'racism' will persist). If social change begins with the individual, let global change begin with our individualizing paradigm, embodied in each analyst who has the constitution to evolve (see Appendix). Our synthetic theory is as a conglomeration of gold seeds from around the globe. It is intrinsically Ours.

Right is of no Sex – Truth is of no Color – God is the Father of us all, and we are all Brethren.

(Douglass 1975)

Acknowledgments

Portions of this book's Introduction and a version of this chapter were previously published in *Journal of Analytical Psychology* (Carter 2021).

Notes

1 Previously published in *Journal of Analytical Psychology*, 2021, 66, I, 70–92.
2 Jung, C. G. (1973). *Letters, Vol. I*, p. 85.
3 Archibald 'Archie' Bunker is a fictional character from two American television sitcoms, *All in the Family* (Lear 1971–1979) and *Archie Bunker's Place* (Lear 1979–1983). Through this character, creator Norman Lear presented a working-class man who struggled with his family over current social issues. Archie's bigotry was often in the spotlight (The Internet Movie Database, www.imdb.com, accessed 2020).
4 The Jungian Psychoanalytic Association with The New School, *Displacements: Inner and Outer*, 2 February 2019.

References

Akbar, N. (1984). *Chains and Images of Psychological Slavery*. Jersey City: New Mind Productions.
Ansley, F.L. (1989). 'Stirring the Ashes: Race, Class and the Future of Civil Rights Scholarship'. *Cornell Law Review*, 74, 993–994. Extracted from 'The Language of White Supremacy: Narrow Definitions of the Term Actually Help Continue the Work of Architects of the Post-Jim Crow Radical Hierarchy', ed. Vann R. Newkirk II. *The Atlantic*. 6 October 2017. https://www.theatlantic.com/politics/archive/2017/10/the-language-of-white-supremacy/542148/
Brewster, F. (2017). *African Americans and Jungian Psychology: Leaving the Shadows*. Abingdon: Routledge.

Brewster, F. (2019). 'Binding Legacies: Ancestor, Archetype and Other'. *Journal of Analytical Psychology*, 64, 3, 306–319.

Carter, C. J. (2021). 'Time for Space at the Table: An African American-Native American Analyst-in-training's First-hand Reflections. A Call for the IAAP to publicly Denounce (But Not Erase) the White Supremacist Writings of C.G. Jung'. *Journal of Analytical Psychology*, 66, I, 70–92.

Cuomo, A. (2020). 'Governor Cuomo Issues Statement Regarding Novel Coronavirus in New York'. 1 March 2020. https://www.governor.ny.gov/news/governor-cuomo-issues-statement-regarding-novel-coronavirus-new-york

Dalal, F. (1988). 'Jung: A Racist'. *British Journal of Psychotherapy*, 4, 263–279.

Douglass, F. (1894). 'The Address by Hon. Fredrick Douglass, Delivered in the Metropolitan A.M.E. Church, Washington, D.C., Tuesday, 9 January 1894, on the Lessons of the Hour, in Which he Discusses the Various Aspects of the So-called, but Mis-called, Negro Problem'. Baltimore: Press of Thomas & Evans.

Douglass, F. (1975). *The Life and Writings of Frederick Douglass: Supplementary Volume 5. 1844–1860*, ed. Philip S. Foner. US: International Publishers.

Du Bois, W.E.B. (1903/1989). *The Souls of Black Folk*. New York: Viking Penguin.

Duvall, T. & Costello, D. (2020). 'Breonna Taylor Was Briefly Alive After Police Shot Her. But No One Tried to Treat Her'. *Louisville Courier Journal*, 17 July 2020.

Fausset, R. (2020). 'What we Know about the Shooting Death of Ahmaud Arbery'. 10 September. https://www.nytimes.com/article/ahmaud-arbery-shooting-georgia.html

Fields, K.E. & Fields, B.J. (2012/2014). *Racecraft: The Soul of Inequality in American Life*. London: Verso.

Hill, E., Tiefenthäler, A., Triebert, C., Jordan, D., Willis, H. & Stein, R. (31 May 2020; 5 November 2020). 'How George Floyd Was Killed in Police Custody'. *The New York Times*. https://www.nytimes.com/2020/05/31/us/george-floyd-investigation.html

Human Rights Watch (12 May 2020). 'Covid-19 Fueling Anti-Asian Racism and Xenophobia Worldwide: National Action Plans Needed to Counter Intolerance'. https://www.hrw.org/news/2020/05/12/covid-19-fueling-anti-asian-racism-and-xenophobia-worldwide

Jung, C.G. (1926). 'Spirit and life'. *Collected Works of C. G. Jung, Vol. 8: Structure & Dynamics of the Psyche*. 2nd Ed. H. Read, M. Fordham, G. Adler and W. McGuire, eds. R. F. C. Hull, Trans. Princeton: Princeton University Press, 1969.

Jung, C.G. (1928). 'Phenomena resulting from the assimilation of the unconscious'. CW 7.

Jung, C.G. (1930). 'The complications of American psychology'. CW 10.

Jung, C.G. (1931). *Visions Vol. 1*. In *Visions: Notes of the Seminar Given in 1930–1934, Vols. 1, 2*, ed. C. Douglas. Princeton: Princeton University Press.

Jung, C.G. (1932). *Visions Vol. 2*. In *Visions: Notes of the Seminar Given in 1930–1934, Vols. 1, 2*, ed. C. Douglas. Princeton: Princeton University Press.

Jung, C.G. (1935). 'Tavistock Lectures II'. *CW* 18.

Jung, C.G. (1939). 'The Symbolic Life (Discussion)'. *CW* 18.

Jung, C.G. (1961/1989). *Memories, Dreams and Reflections*, ed. A. Jaffé. New York: Random House, Inc.

Jung, C.G. (1973). *Letters, Volume 1, 1906–1950*, ed. G. Adler, trans. R.F.C. Hull. Princeton, NJ: Princeton University Press.

Jung, C.G. (2009). *The Red Book. Liber Novus, A Reader's Edition*, ed. S. Shamdasani. New York & London: W.W. Norton.

Kennedy, R.F. (2013). 'Introduction'. *Race and Ethnicity in the Classical World: An Anthology of Primary Sources in Translation*. Indianapolis: Hackett Publishing Company.

Lear, N. (Developer). (1971–1979). *All in the Family*. [Television series]. Hollywood: CBS Television.

Lear, N. (Developer). (1979–1983). *Archie Bunker's Place*. [Television series]. Hollywood: CBS Television.

Mehrtens, S. (2014). Blog, 28 September: 'Jung on the Provisional Life'. https://jungiancenter.org/jung-on-the-provisional-life/

Morgan, H. (2004). 'Exploring Racism'. *The Cultural Complex: Contemporary Jungian Perspectives on Psyche and Society*, eds. T. Singer & S.L. Kimbles. New York: Brunner-Routledge.

Oppel Jr., R.A., Taylor, D.B. & Bogel-Burroughs, N. (30 Oct 2020). 'What to Know About Breonna Taylor's Death: Fury over the Killing of Ms. Taylor by the Police Fueled Tense Demonstrations in Louisville, Ky., and Elsewhere'. *The New York Times*. https://www.nytimes.com/article/breonna-taylor-police.html

Powell, D.R. (2018). 'Race, African Americans, and Psychoanalysis: Collective Silence in the Therapeutic Conversation', 1 December. *Journal of the American Psychological Association*, 66, 6, 1021–1049.

Richards, G. (1997). *'Race', Racism and Psychology: Towards a Reflexive History*. New London: Routledge.

Terry, W.S. (2008). 'A Missed Opportunity for Psychology: The Story of Solomon Carter Fuller'. *Association for Psychological Science: Observer*, June/July (1 June 2008).

The Internet Movie Database. *All in the Family*. https://www.imdb.com/title/tt0066626/

The Internet Movie Database. *Archie Bunker's Place*. https://www.imdb.com/title/tt0078562/

Ulanov, A.B. (2014). *Knots and their Untying: Essays on Psychological Dilemmas*. New Orleans: Spring Journal Books.

United Nations Education, Scientific and Cultural Organization (1950). 'The Race Question'. *UNESCO and its Programme*, 3 [31]. Paris: UNESCO[24241]. https://unesdoc.unesco.org/ark:/48223/pf0000128291

Vaughan, A.G. (2019). 'African American Cultural History and Reflections on Jung in the African Diaspora'. *Journal of Analytical Psychology*, 64, 3, 320–348.

Woodson, C.G. (1931). 'The Miseducation of the Negro'. *The Crisis*. August 1931, 266.

Appendix

A Call for the International Association for Analytical Psychology to Take Corrective Actions, Publicly Denunciating (But Not Erasing) the White Supremacist Writings of Carl Gustav Jung

Christopher Jerome Carter

According to Jung, 'You know no Negro can bear to be stared at, all primitives instantly look away, because one might cast the evil eye on them. The Pueblo Indians always turn their eyes away, and Negroes are particularly shifty' (Jung 1932, p. 620). I am grateful that the IAAP has a non-discrimination policy. This policy does not absolve the IAAP from the responsibility of publishing a unified statement that publicly denounces the racist writings of Jung (not to be misconstrued as the totality of his work). Corrective actions are overdue, both on local and international levels. The initial next step would be to express remorse for ways our collective attitude may have excluded others. This is not to delay the IAAP from making a public statement. The Jungian Psychoanalytic Association (JPA) has lost a candidate of color partially due to tendencies to defend Jung's bigotry. I have analysands who are wrestling with Jung now, having done their research privately. They ask, 'Why do you want to be a Jungian?' I was admonished and questioned by brilliant scholars, descendants of the African diaspora and others. I was reading *Visions* while riding the subway from the Bronx to the JPA Treatment Center in Manhattan when an apparently homeless Black male asked, in shock, 'Are you reading Jung?!' People of color are more familiar with Jung than others tend to believe. The theory is extracted from the greater collective and belongs to us all. In expressing our remorse and skewing from Jung's racist and misogynist barbs, we remove the fences that were established through Jung's personal and social misgivings.

In the Open Letter, many analysts offered signatures of support for training institutes and all involved in analytical psychology to accept responsibility for fostering real steps in addressing the harm that has been supported by, and is the result of decades of unaddressed errors. However, it is time for the IAAP to take real steps in denouncing Jung's racist writings. I do not promote erasing his views. But the IAAP has an unacknowledged responsibility to take real action in opening-up the value of our paradigm to all who have the constitution to benefit from it. I propose that the IAAP communicates in writing that:

1 The IAAP denounces the aspects of Jung's work that are racist and misogynist as detrimental and peripheral to analytic theory, which is about the differentiation and the relationship of opposing energies, and inclusivity toward the enlargement of the personality.

2 The IAAP expresses regret for the harmful impact that may have foreclosed opportunities to collaborate with other psychoanalytic paradigms in theoretical development toward alleviating emotional distress and mental illnesses.

3 The IAAP supports analytic training institutes with increased attention to the impact of bias, prejudice, and 'diversity'. The IAAP supports increased attention to transcultural and intercultural perspectives and knowledge, as reflected in the curriculum and public seminars of analytic training institutes.

These corrective actions, along with such announcements in public forums, will allow others to read and hear that our theory proposes the betterment of society at large through the healing of each person, as a unique individual. In doing so, the IAAP and individuals may actively promote greater inclusivity to prospective Black and Brown analysts while simultaneously promoting an increase in collaborations with other psychoanalytic paradigms – collaborations long-delayed because of matters conveyed by Jung that are not integral to analysis. We expand by acknowledging that Jung, a very gifted man, was also flawed. Everyone has limits. Individuation is an ongoing process, occurring by degrees. 'The term "race" came into existence at a discernible historical moment for rationally understandable historical reasons and is subject to change for similar reasons' (Fields & Fields 2012/2014, p. 121). Together, we can educate those within our reach to withdraw from the harmful ideology of race (although racism and racists will persist).

References

Fields, K.E. & Fields, B.J. (2012/2014). *Racecraft: The Soul of Inequality in American Life*. London: Verso.

Jung, C.G. (1932). *Visions: Notes of the Seminar Given in 1930–1934*, Vol. 2, ed. C. Douglas. Princeton: Princeton University Press (1997).

'Open Letter from a Group of Jungians on the Question of Jung's Writings on and Theories about "Africans"'. (2018). *British Journal of Psychotherapy*, 34, 4, 673–678.

Chapter 2

The Paradox of the Primitive and Jung's Relation to 'Negroes'

Ann Ulanov

The murder of George Floyd (25 May 2020; Minneapolis, Minnesota) opened wider the racial wound of whites against Blacks in America. It went viral, like another pandemic, because a woman of seventeen captured it on her phone. Crimes against Blacks were no longer 'elsewhere', in some other city. Elsewhere was here, now, in our personal and collective consciousness. We changed from observers to participants. A man on radio news said, 'I saw my father's face, my brother's, my face under the cop's knee'.

This calamity moved psychoanalysts to get more conscious of white supremacy and the systemic nature of racism and to address their effects on clinical work and in training students, those of color and those of no color. I joined such a group. We noted Jung's remarks about 'Negroes'—some expressing bluntly or implied racism, some expressing kinship and admiration.[1]

My approach is to set the issue of Jung's relation to Negroes in the larger scene of Jung's relation to the primitive. He places the American and African negro in that context. It is important to note here in the beginning that, as far as I can find, Jung had no close personal relation with an educated, cultured black person, or a collegial relation with a black psychiatrist, nor a connection with any of the black geniuses of his time. He identified the lack with the primitive man (with brief mention of his observations of the strict separation of women from the men during his travels though Africa).

Jung is ambivalent about primitive. His descriptions of it as a state of mind alternates back and forth between negative and positive. That alternation yields to paradox.

Primitive as negative

Jung emphasizes that the primitive layer of psyche exists in all of us and it is vitally important for the individual and the world. In the primitive layer of our psychology, subject and object are identified. No space yet exists between subject and object, so there is not yet perception of self as separate from the object. In the primitive layer of psyche, there is no perception of the object as separate from the self's unconscious projections onto the object. Psyche and

DOI: 10.4324/9781003311447-3

object are identified. We perceive through our projections at this primitive layer of psyche. Neither symbol of affect nor of a quality also found in the object is yet available. As symbols arise from the psychic depths into ego consciousness, they make spaces between subject and object. Symbols make spaces between the outer object and the inner image, stirred by the libido that is somewhat drained from the object and returned to the subject which awakens such primordial images in our psyche. This space, slim as it may be, allows us a tiny margin of choice and the emerging perception that we help construct the object we see, and that we help build the meaning we find (Jung 1921, paras 414, 422, 425).

The power of a life force or mana or God or fetish object 'resides in the libido which is present in the subject's unconscious, and is perceived in the object because wherever unconscious contents are activated they appear in projection' (Jung 1921, para. 414). The libido can go back and forth as in the primitives' sense of their soul, yet the soul lives in a leopard in the bush. When the libido flows back into the primitive subject, it stirs the unconscious, which awakens primitive images within the subject. Symbol arises when a space emerges between subject and object; they begin to be experienced as differentiated. The primitive concretizes, the civilized symbolizes.

Jung applies these negative aspects of the primitive to Negroes, reducing the specific person to an abstract category of 'primitive'. Their thinking is through projecting. Hence, they lack objective evaluation of differences between what is *there* in the other and what is *here* in me. Jung likens the primitive's mind to a child's in which inner and outer suffuse each other. Jung judges the primitive pejoratively as being less developed and inferior to scientific rational and empirical reasoning (Jung 1921, para. 12).

Paradoxically, Jung says we can only reach more objective knowledge if we acknowledge the part our subjectivity plays in constructing it. We must depsychologize our knowing if we want to reach some objective psychology, by seeing how much we project our unconscious into the act of constructing knowledge. The way to do this is to become aware of our 'personal equation'. We must accept that we see both objectively *and* subjectively—never only objectively. As in physics, the stance of the observer influences what is observed. Our personal equation includes what we are still unconscious and hence project into the object, our personal style and limits, and our ability (or lack thereof) to form our view in communicable terms, accepting it has validity but never total 'rightness'. Unlike the primitive, we see our projections to some degree though we also remain unconscious of many of them (Jung 1921, para. 9; Ulanov 2015, pp. 167–72).

The primitive lacks ability for such self-awareness and cannot yet see what is there objectively in the object, differentiated from what they project onto the object. Acknowledging our personal equation depends on becoming an individual capable of distinguishing between what is conscious and unconscious, what is self and what is other, what is my projection and what is the object in itself as different from me. Jung avers that the primitive lacks this capacity entirely, has not achieved a self-conscious, individual perspective, in fact, is like any animal in the collective unconscious.

Here Jung links primitive with his formulation of the collective unconscious. I suggest that this linking causes mix-ups and needs distinction. Jung writes,

> if we go back into history ... right back to primitive psychology, we find absolutely no trace of the concept of the individual. Instead of individuality we find ... the mind that is quite incapable of thinking and feeling in any other way than by projection.
>
> (Jung 1921, para. 12)

To see our projections, we must have some space of separation of subject from other—of subject from object—instead of knowledge 'filled with projected psychology'. It is in this sense that we need to de-psychologize psychology to construct a psychology that can communicate objective things about the human psyche that apply to all of us.

I disagree with this notion that 'no self at all' existed in early times. Surely Jung is correct in pointing out big differences between modern and earliest times in what was understood by individual, but to say no such self existed then communicates, I suggest, something else entirely that forms what I call a 'collective equation'.

Like the personal equation, the collective equation means we are unconsciously identified with our society's collective viewpoint. Like the personal equation but now on a general level applied to the whole society, we spy the mote in the eye of another group or even a whole culture but miss what is missing or wrong in our group's or our culture's perception—the elusive beam that belongs to us. Thus, objectivity escapes us until we also take into account that our views, personal and collective, are partial, never totally definitive.

Jung is in company of the best thinkers (except Franz Boas, who disagrees) in this idea that no individual sense existed before we moderns. Identifying the individual with consciousness that Jung defines as differentiation seems to me to be full of collective projections onto the early past and onto present-day Negroes, who Jung lumps into primitive. Mixed in with the capacity to perceive difference and differentiation (e.g., words versus pictures, thoughts versus smells, reason versus emotion) is judgement of a pejorative nature of 'less than', 'inferior to'. The projection carries a whiff of fear of otherness as the individual in primitive groups is surely differently conjugated in contrast to the modern emphasis on separation of subject and object, which too often turns into hierarchical labeling of more and less—more developed and less so, more rational and lacking reason, more progress-oriented and none at all.

That view has always struck me as masking fear, but of what? Perhaps of engulfment by something so different it threatens to overwhelm. Evidence has emerged of a different point of view. What are we to make, for example, of a prehistoric cave painting that asserts the opposite of total lack of individuality? The cave painting shows a handprint distinguished from many others by a distinct detail of a pinkie finger with a kink in it. It almost shouts, "Here I am!" The hand has a characteristic that identifies it, scholars surmise, as belonging to a unique individual, probably six feet tall, male, existing $32,000^{+/-}$ years ago (Chauvet-Pont d'Arc Cave of southern France). This detail of the cave painting's distinguishing finger does not comply with Jung's use of Lucien Levy-Bruhl's idea of *participation mystique* to assert that primitives lived collective relationships immersed in an archetypal, unconscious layer of psyche and incapable of thinking and feeling in a personal, individual way (Jung 1931/1964, paras 130–31, 134–35). A sense of individual and other may simply conjugate differently from binary conscious terms of the 'civilized' human being. In this notion of the primitive having no self, I suggest, Jung was embedded in the collective equation of his times without being conscious of it.

We also are amazed by the primitive artist's respect and clarity about the distinct other creatures in the cave paintings—the antelope, mammoth, deer, horse, bull so notably alive, as if moving legs cantering across the walls. We see this same acuity in contemporary Aboriginal women painters who give their individual signature mark to their paintings of cosmos, land, sky, which simultaneously displays their linking to community. These are works not of a nonself but of an extraordinarily awake self to the surroundings in which they paint their anchoring (Skeritt 2016, pp. 62, 91, 120–21).

An example of individuality and togetherness of the primitive in and by Negroes may go a long way to underscore there was a self differently registered in the past. Evidence of a diverse conjugation of self and other is found in the creation of jazz, where black musicians abound. Here improvisation is central to each musician playing a solo and even a chatting back and forth between two instruments as if in conversation as they go round to include dissimilar sounds and rhythms in each player's solo. Then the climax of all differing ones playing together creates a unity of diversity that also is originary. It can be repeatedly improvised but cannot be imitated. That creativeness making the spontaneous new sound arouses hope in the hearers, the jazz lovers. How else except with this detail of immense individual assertion could a whole people show resilience against the slavery inflicted for hundreds of years, having been sold as objects, as though commodities to further those who could and therefore did enslave Africans and descendants of Africans in America for their own profit, greed, and to quell their fear? The danger of remaining unconscious of collective equations is shown precisely in the fear of difference transmogrifying into *concepts* of the "inferior race" to justify shameless exploitation of others in every possible way erasing them in order to profit financially, legally, sadistically.

The primitive as positive

Jung's recognition of the positive of the primitive layer of psyche is robust and detailed. More significantly, it is there in our psyche, and we need it. The primitive is the 'taproot' of our psyche, connecting us to the ever-present fountainhead of the unconscious. Yes, its danger is that it can overwhelm our ego and interrupt the conscious identity that marks our individuality. But without living communication with this taproot, we fall into deadness, including loss of soul. The 'archaic man' projects his unconscious contents 'through *participation mystique* ... psychic happenings are projected so completely that they cannot be distinguished from objective physical events' (Jung 1931/1964, para. 135). He brings about a world completely psychically contained by identification through projection. He does not dominate nature but submits to its chance happenings, to 'arbitrary and intentional acts, interventions by animate beings' (ibid.). He does not see the factor of his own projections into the animation of those outside beings. They have their souls, which are concrete objects located somewhere else. All things have soul, but he does not, and Jung remarks how pivotal the ceremony of baptism is, endowing the individual 'with a living soul, lifting him out of his identification with the world into a being who stands above it ... the birth of the spiritual man who transcends nature' (ibid., para. 136).

Jung surmises that the paradoxical also happens. The primitive is concerned with the nexus point between, 'Do we create beauty with our own astonishment and fear', or 'Does its mana reside in the concrete object, the thing's beauty that compels our response?' (ibid., paras 136, 139)? Jung says, 'Archaic man believes it to be the sun, and civilized man believes it to be the eye. The primitive must take back all his projections in order to see the world objectively' (ibid., para. 135). For him all psychic life is concrete and objective. For us our theory that unconscious life is automatically projected outward, a portion of the psyche 'has the character of personality, is personified ... . Whenever an autonomous component of the psyche is projected, an invisible person comes into being' (ibid., para. 137). Thus emerges the primitive's belief in spirits, or voices of the insane, or the mana personality gets constructed. The village woman has a soul, but it is a leopard living in the bush. There is some power called mana that may migrate into a person. This means a paradox for the primitive: objects and their power are only objective, not invested by me, yet some mysterious energy existing in the outside world also does invest in the object. Jung asserts, 'Being is a field of force. The primitive idea of mana ... has in it the beginnings of a crude theory of energy' (ibid., para. 139).

I focus on the both/and quality of the primitive gifting us with an intensely valuable asset, especially with contemporary concerns with climate change and efforts to cooperate with nature lest we destroy our planet by continuing to dominate it. Might we say this gift of the primitive perspective includes our experiences of looking upon nature and creation looking upon itself.

This evokes an inner experience as well as an outer experience of beauty. Musicians speak of getting inside music and playing it from there, inside-out, from spaces between notes as well as hitting the perfect tonal pitch. Dancers might say the same about movement or painters trying to capture that indefinable meeting of what is there and my experience of what is there. Physicists, engineers, caretakers of children, gardeners, cooks know of this nexus point where we create what we find and find what we create (Ulanov 2020, Chapter 8).

Jung notes positive factors of the primitive mind. When we are not viewing them from our identification with our contemporary consciousness as the superior goal to achieve, these traits and skills elicit wonder. We hope to teach our analysts-in-training such skills. Jung finds in the primitive mind his notion of the imago (that image that combines what is there in the object with what we project onto the object): 'the psychic reverberation of the sense-perception, so strong and so sensuously coloured that when it is reproduced as a spontaneous memory-image it sometimes even has the quality of a hallucination' (Jung 1931/ 1964, para. 46). Whereas we think about the dead, the primitive actually perceives them because 'of the extraordinary sensuousness of his mental images ... thought is visionary and auditory, hence it has the character of a revelation' (ibid.).

Although the primitive on the negative side mistakes the psychic for the real, on the positive side, his perspective adds another way of perceiving, likened to artists of all kinds, to intuitives, sensates and mystics. Jung comments, 'The instinctive sensuousness of the primitive has its counterpart in the spontaneity of his psychic processes: his mental products, his thoughts, just appear to him ... . It is not he ... who thinks them ... they happen to him' (ibid., para. 254). The painter Clyfford Still said the new vertical images that changed all his subsequent painting just appeared and he spent the rest of his life trying to understand them (Clyfford Still Museum - Denver). Bion talks of thoughts that arrive to the thinker who did not make them. Jung has the same instruction from Philemon, the Self figure of *The Red Book*, that your thoughts happen; you do not invent them. That kind of experience is dramatized by the playwright Luigi Pirandello in *Six Characters in Search of an Author*. Religious geniuses speak of God speaking to them, and mystics 'endeavor to recapture the primitive reality of the image' (Jung 1921/1971, para. 47). In Jungian training, there is emphasis on the fact of the image *per se* bespeaking psychic reality in addition to gathering personal and cultural associations from the context of the dream or symptom, indicating that the image has its independent verity in addition to what we make of it (Ulanov 2022, Chapter 1).

Jung saw primitive bearers, hunters, chiefs as having entirely different presuppositions than–Europeans, attributing to sorcery, magic, or chance the cause of things just as we would refer to natural causes. As Jung puts it, 'His mental functioning does not differ in any fundamental way from ours. It is ... his assumptions alone that distinguish him from ourselves'

(Jung 1931/1964, para. 107). His morality about good and evil is just as good as ours, only different in the forms under which they occur. There are loyal head-hunters, as there are those who do 'cruel rites, or murder from sacred conviction ... the process of ethical judgement is the same' (ibid., para. 108). Toward things outside their experience, they 'are slow and clumsy' and prolonged mental activity like serious conversation for more than two hours fatigues them, but toward travels within their country, primitives are as 'keen-sighted as hawks', with 'incredibly accurate sense of direction', 'astonishing concentration and endurance', 'strong powers of observation' (ibid., paras 109–11).

Fear and kinship

These positive and negative aspects of the primitive mind exist simultaneously together in this level of psyche, and it exists in all of us (Jung 1930/1939/1976, para. 1288; Jung 1931/1964, para. 105). Jung sees the primitive layer of psyche closer to the surface in the black person, implying less development personally and culturally, whereas the white has that additional historical layer of culture, hence more developed, but also more distant from the tap-root found in the primitive layer (Jung 1939/1976, para. 93; Jung 1930/1939/1976, para. 1288). The white must reach to the primitive way down in the unconscious; hence he is in danger of lacking connection to it. The white must make connection to the primitive layer with consciousness, to experience its interpenetration with his identity lest he go dead in stultified cultural customs.

Jung remembers an American dinner with adults that he finds so constricting, he is compelled to tell jokes which fails to rouse humor in his hosts! They stiffen instead. But then Jung feels freed and pleasure when behind him from a young Black American waiter 'an avalanche of laughter broke loose'. Recalling it, Jung exclaims, 'How I loved that African brother' (Jung 1931/1964, para. 950).

When talking about the centrality of dreams in any process of individuation (coming to be all of who one is), Jung also exclaims that he, just like the Negro, is dependent on his dreaming (Jung 1939/1976, para. 674). However, Jung uses the now shunned n-word that exerts a shock on the reader. The editors provide a footnote that disavows the term's racist impact, saying this was not a derogatory term at the time that Jung wrote it. This suggests to me the collective equation at work. Calling the other disparaging names speaks an assumption they are not the same as us, but less than. We erase them as mutual citizens and construct theories of race to justify doing so. For students in class, it would be crucial to note such derogatory language and to make space to feel the negative impact of such dismissal. To ignore it erases the erasure and the harm done.

Jung recognizes that the harm whites have done to Blacks is legion. Such events elicit the primitive in everyone in the class, which is unconscious, which means the content is automatically projected into the teaching field. The class crowds up. An unconscious content first makes itself known in projection. Class members may experience the interpenetration of primitive and civilized right there in themselves. In such an intense moment, something can happen and change your life.

Jung shows both negative and positive views of the primitive and of Negroes he places there. Along with sharing the laughter, Jung appreciates what he saw as the Negroes' pleasure of motility, expressive emotionality, 'loose-jointed walk ... dancing and music ... . American music is most obviously pervaded by the African rhythm and the African melody' (ibid., para. 964). We get both kinship and fear in the remarks Jung makes about Blacks.

Jung in blackness

In the face of the primitive, even with its taproot of the psyche, Jung dreaded disorientation, loss of civilized, developed parts of himself. He felt the negative and positive of the primitive but not together simultaneously as in a paradox with the strain of holding both in consciousness at the same time, from which might emerge a reconciling transcendent function.

In Jung's depiction of the primitive, the opposites of negative and positive stayed in an alternating rhythm. His dread of the negative came in different forms. In one, he observes America as a country of Blacks and whites, yet the majority still stayed with the latter. If America should fall under the majority of blackness, then the danger of contagion could happen. Here, the mix-up of collective unconscious and the primitive causes confusion from which flows prejudice and discrimination. Jung places Negroes in the primitive and identifies them with it. He places the primitive in the collective unconscious. Jung was still experiencing these phenomena; they emerge from the primary material of *The Red and Black Books*. More differentiation of these psychic dimensions develops.

I suggest that the primitive is an aspect of the collective unconscious, but not defined by it. If there is lesion in the ego or a burgeoning part of the collective unconscious, it invades like a big wave that can wash away the personal ego and the guidelines of collective consciousness (e.g., weakening restraints against screaming in a school class, or against rageful outbursts in society). As representing the primitive in Jung's fear, Blacks could overwhelm whites. That fear seeps in unconsciously. The bursting out of white supremacy again in the twenty-first century shows the mountains of denied fear of this very either/or threat of who is in the majority, as if fighting for their lives and hence killing those who threaten to become the majority. The possibility of all of us (as a people) of both/and is unimaginable. To accept blackness is to feel whiteness extinguished. Hence the murderous reaction.

Jung links the Negro with living in the collective unconscious, not yet having a personal feeling or thought (Jung 1931/1964, paras 128, 130, 132).

Jung notes the significance that when in Africa, he never dreams of Africa, which makes him conclude Africa is not yet real to him but existing on a symbolic level. He cites a pivotal dream that displays his terror of the threat of losing his European civilized identity. He dreams he is in the chair of his Black barber from Tennessee of twelve years ago who puts a hot curling iron to his hair 'to give me Negro hair. I could already feel the painful heat, and awoke with a sense of terror … the primitive is a danger to me' (Jung 1961/1963, p. 274).

I was struck by hair being the central symbol of the danger of 'going Black' (ibid., p. 272). Hair grows autonomously, even after death, and has been seen as representing creative thoughts, ideas, images, intuitions. Jung writes of being in the grip of the daimon creativeness that gives him no choice but to follow, despite hurting others whom he leaves when they do not feed this spirit (ibid., pp. 356–57). He works throughout his life, from earliest childhood to recollections, before dying to bring into communicable forms the new that shows itself to him. Throughout *The Red Book* and *The Black Books*, he ever seeks to 'understand', to get the 'meaning of', and he is chastised by the soul just to let psychic events happen. To have 'Negro hair' enforced upon him is to succumb to the primitive, losing the creativeness central to his identity. Primitivity means the loss of his personal European, civilized self that could affect a connection to the taproot, to the Self, not be obliterated by it. Hair may be seen as representing creative thought, and Jung was full of ideas of an originary nature.

A third danger is in Jung's use of the primitive to bolster his theory of the collective unconscious. When hearing of a burning wheel image in the dream of a Black man in a psychiatric hospital in Washington D.C., Jung saw that image as relating to archetypal imagery (Ixion) and thus giving evidence that despite differences between black and white and of people in or out of mental hospitals, at a depth level we all share a taproot of primordial images *qua* being human. The limits of this dream interpretation are ably criticized and expanded, showing its cultural and personal roots by Brewster and Morgan, leaving the reader with a larger perspective of multi-views (Morgan 2021, p. 78; Brewster 2013).

Jung was enamored by the collective unconscious and took the archetypal wheel image as evidence of the immortal in us, that endures while the personal wanes. Jung is careful also to say that this is our experience of the immortal; we do not know the immortal in itself. Here he forgot his insistence on knowing the total situation of the dreamer, not just the symbol. He subsumed the dreamer's wheel into his new idea of collective unconscious and did not take account of the possible negative personal and cultural links for the dreamer of the burning wheel as an instrument of torture of Blacks and/or as positive for Blacks of religious revelation of God.

Jung says we must go back to the barbarian in us to secure the soul's place, to the force of it in us, if we are to go forward. This takes us to the shadow as well as collective unconscious because soul says she can be lured to evil, to shiny frauds, instead of the real thing (Jung 1913–1932/2020 v. 6, p. 286). This happens to her when she does not trust Jung to entrust himself to the light within him: 'Light that is no knowledge, but—fact' (ibid., v. 7, p. 216). Barbarism and loss of soul go together, the former to be accepted, the latter to be secured. Black people give us routes to the positive and negative primitive in ourselves, says Jung. But most times Jung alternates between positive and negative, not holding their tension consciously together, experienced as paradox.

Blackness in Jung

Despite Jung's racist remarks which he does not clean up nor flaunt, it is a surprise to read the remarkable experiences he has of feeling led toward wholeness through Black figures in his imagination and his dreams. They are of great value to him; he honors their meaning. Jung's psyche presents them to him as harbingers of Self, the central concept of his work that emerges from his *Red Book* and *Black Books* journeys.

Near the beginning of *The Red Book*, a shortish brown man aids Jung in killing Siegfried. Looking back, Jung realizes this brown man is a Self figure that joins in slaying of the dominance of his superior function of thinking and the hero complex Siegfried symbolizes (Jung 2009, pp. 241–42). Jung sacrifices his identification with this function as superior and opens to meeting his incapacity—the inferior function of feeling, left to moral decay within himself (ibid., pp. 264, 366).

A second example, from Jung's first trip to Africa in 1920 (Jung 1961/1963, p. 238), includes an aristocratic dark man who passes Jung travelling to the oasis of Nefta. 'Swathed in white', with 'proud bearing', who passed by with no greetings, 'an elegant, impressive figure', as if outside of time— 'unselfconsciously the person he had always been' in contrast to the European who feels 'something has been taken from him' and hence is 'incomplete' which 'he compensates for by the illusion of his triumphs' (ibid., p. 240). Following his insight that the primitive man lives from his affects and emotions without reflection, highlighting that the civilized European lacks such 'intensity of life', Jung dreams he is in an Arab city crossing a bridge to the inside of a mandala-shaped casbah. Halfway across the bridge to enter the citadel, 'a handsome, dark, Arab of … almost royal bearing … the prince of the citadel' and the 'double of the proud Arab who had ridden past … without a greeting', attacks Jung and tries to kill him. They fight and burst through the bridge railing, fall into the waters of the moat below, and each tries to drown the other. Jung wins. He pushes the dark man's head under water in order not to be killed himself, not because he wanted to kill the dark one (ibid., pp. 243–44).

Then the dark one becomes a boy. This boy is the double of the proud Arab who had snubbed Jung, passing by without a greeting. Jung experiences this boy as 'an emissary of the self'. Recalling Jacob's fight with the angel, Jung feels this boy is such an angel who needs to learn about humans, just as Jung needs to learn about the angel-boy whose departure point is so contrary to his own.

Jung had attempted to suppress this dark primitive that tried to kill him, but his subconscious put it forward as belonging to himself, seeing this 'Arab's dusky complexion marks him as a "shadow" but not the personal shadow, rather the ethnic one associated not with my persona but with the totality of my personality ... with the self' (ibid., pp. 244–45). Here is Jung facing blackness within him, 'the shadow of the self' (ibid.). 'I was not prepared for the existence of unconscious forces within myself that would take the part of these strangers with such intensity' expressed 'in the symbol of an attempted murder' (ibid., pp. 243–45).

This danger for the 'uprooted European in Africa' of being changed by the primitive within appears again in Jung's second trip to Africa in 1925 (ibid., p. 253). He discovers he belongs with the primitive in his personality, conscious of blackness that is *his*, not automatically projected onto Blacks.

The appearance of murderous conflict calls to mind two other occasions when Jung acknowledges such aggression. In 1923, a shade sheathed in death says Jung overcame him, a God, but Jung does not know it. He seeks Jung to get actual human beingness for himself. Jung is filled with dread, terror. Hearing this god whistle for his hounds 'freezes the blood' (Jung 1913–1932/ 2020 v. 7, p. 228). 'I had to defend my life, even if a God attacked' (ibid., p. 229). Yet Jung recognizes this force of life as a master, the maker of terrible riddles and identifies him with the Arab man of this Africa dream (ibid., p. 227). Jung links this terrific force to the 'God who comes', saying, 'when he came, he was shockingly new. I confess I am stunned ... a God of fear and ruthless obedience, a fool with a lightning hammer ... . But a man, a master, a mighty one! It's a pleasure to obey him' (ibid., p. 230). Despite his tremendous power, this God consents to learn from Jung the wisdom of 'right action that is in accord with the whole and the whole leads to greater life ... wisdom destroys unjust power and gives form to right power' (ibid., p. 229).

This conflict of a murderous, aggressive force with the necessity to learn wisdom comes up in a later seminar (1932) in a woman's vision of going down into the deepest hold in a ship, seeing a man reading a book of illumination on the wisdom of Tao and seeing many Negroes in chains (Jung 1932/1997 v. 2, p. 678). She asks why the man does not liberate them from this cruelty. He ignores her and reads his book. Jung explains she cannot attain Tao if the Negroes are freed. They represent repressed instincts, the chained up primitive in herself. If let loose, she cannot reach the stillness needed to learn wisdom, for one cannot be told about Tao; 'one must experience it to understand' (ibid.). 'She could not possibly experience Tao if her primordial instincts were around loose on all sides ... . To have the experience the instincts must first be chained' (ibid.), and Jung adds, 'Naturally every human being is trying to do something about those chained Negroes ... they must be liberated' (ibid., p. 681).

The problem is that Negroes here are reduced to symbols of what needs to be restrained, locked up cruelly, the negative primitive, the invading collective unconscious which would destroy the ego. To let them loose right away before Tao is experienced creates 'great turmoil' (ibid., p. 680). We spread our problem of not knowing these instincts over everyone, and then we meet that problem with what ought to be done to solve it, but it is no longer our own, but everyone's: 'It becomes *participation mystique* which spreads out all over the world; you infect everybody with your inferiority, your own defects and it does no good whatsoever' (ibid., p. 681). She thinks she is giving compassion, but in fact we are pleasing ourselves with our wonderful kindness, indulging our 'autoerotic pleasure'. 'Those Negroes are murderous devils, who might kill other people as well as yourself, so why should they be free?' (ibid.). The implied meaning, I suggest, is we must reckon with destructive aggression, withdraw to stillness and then to hearing the wisdom of Lao Tzu to sort it in ourselves, using the energy of the primitive as it becomes available to us.

Jung takes this further. We must 'love inside out', give energy, love, to our inferior sides, not let them loose in the disguise of helping others (Jung 1913–32/2020 v. 5, p. 207). The context here of this shocking statement about Negroes as carriers of this fierce energy reduces real live people to a symbol of a killing destructiveness. The collective equation mixes up the symbolic with the concrete. Negroes have a life as a people and a right to live it and cannot be hijacked to be a symbol for whites' or humans' murderous aggression. The collective equation does not sustain firm differentiation of symbolic and concrete lived life, but equates the two at the expense, here, of Blacks. This mix-up obscures the issue facing the woman in her vision and wreaks havoc on living people.

In her vision, Negroes are called 'wild masculinity' symbolizing fierce energy opposite to conventions about femininity in her culture. Investigation and understanding of that conflict and the necessity to develop spiritual muscle to manage murderous aggression and not act out on herself or on others needs further development.

The use of Negroes to symbolize murderous aggression bespeaks, I suggest, the collective equation that subsumed Jung and his time, but maybe not the woman who provided the vision. Her vision touches on 'primitive instincts' locked up in women by their culture and condemned as fearsome, harkening to Erich Neuman's image of the 'masculine' in the Great Mother symbol. We need wisdom, first to handle this great energy, and then to release it in livable forms, not in killing outbursts projected onto and identified with Black men.

This theme of giving energy to inferior parts of ourselves just as we must with the primitive in us Jung addresses in another shocking text. We must 'Love inside out ... . Love the generosity of the miser, the ugly of the beautiful, the rationality of the crazy and the badness of the good' (Jung 1913–1932/2020 v. 5, p. 207). If you want to learn wisdom then deal with untamed 'wild' primitive in you by withdrawing into yourself to improve and be illuminated by a kind of truth that comes from nature, from the unconscious which communicates in images 'not directed thoughts and abstractions constructed by a purposeful mind, they are revelations of nature' (Jung 1932/1997 v. 2, p. 682).

Coming to terms with murderous aggression touches on Jung's personal problem too, I suggest. Jung survived by not letting the Arab dream man kill him, and by overcoming the God whistling for hounds to take a soul to death, but Jung does not know he did that; it is not conscious. And Jung projects the murderous affect that is primitive, unassimilated aggression onto Negroes.

The soul harangues Jung for lacking self-esteem and thus being 'laughably sensitive', (ibid. v. 5, p. 217, 46n), full of 'childish pride', 'craving for power', 'desire for esteem' (ibid., 47n), with 'kindergarten feelings' (ibid. v. 5, p. 222). Ka and Philemon, representing the Self, harangue Jung for not trusting his strength. It remains too unconscious and then gets projected outward in envious ambition, larding his lectures with quotations to show off his superior intellect. He must claim this force, this spark of life, this light inside him, of truth that he discovers by living it. Ka who makes all things real (in actuality, not in angel-land) chides, stop whining, do your work. Your work is the thing. If you do not claim the light in yourself who else will be able to claim this force in their selves (ibid. v. 7, pp. 196, 198)?

Struggling to accept this, Jung discovers the direction of his path: neither to identify with the gods as he sees Christ, Buddha, Mani and Mohamad doing, nor to fall into unconsciousness, nor to found a new church. Jung claims his work, puts it into the world and then retires to his garden. That means housing a seed of the lifeforce in his human self that is a tiny grain of sand (ibid. v. 7, p. 173), an obdurate, primordial kernel, accepting the taproot made available to him in the originary material of his experience. From it, his work is born (his 'son'). Jung is told 'No longer are you an I, but a river that pours forth over the lands' (ibid. v. 6, p. 231). 'Your work is your son, get to work; it will thrive and you will wane' (ibid. v. 4, p. 269; v. 6, p. 265). 'If the Self unfolds, the I shrinks' (ibid. v. 7, p. 248). Jung retired to paint and sculpt in his primitive Bollingen tower, without electricity or plumbing.

Jung expresses the paradox of his own nature: 'Yes, the truth is in me … . The second principle of my truth goes: I don't know' (ibid. v. 7, p. 171). George Bright, in his excellent review of Jung's *The Black Books*, notes the shift of 'the ethical impact of the pursuit of wholeness rather than goodness in personal and social relationships' (Bright 2021, p. 770).

The dark Arab, the attacker in the dream, becomes a boy and he and Jung are inside the citadel. There is a book Jung had written in a foreign tongue that he insists the boy read, despite the boy's resistance. Jung is the 'master of the citadel and the boy must "learn to know man"' (Jung 1961/1963, pp. 240–46).

The two belong together and the suppressed primitive comes to the fore to be learned, lived: 'In the living psychic structure ... everything fits into the economy of the whole' (ibid., p. 246).

The third example of blackness in Jung is the tall thin Black man with a long spear, standing on a cliff top as Jung's train circles below it. This happens 'at the first ray of sunlight ... . On a jagged rock above us a slim, brownish-black figure stood motionless, leaning on a long spear, looking down at the train' (ibid., p. 254). Jung is deeply moved by seeing something 'utterly alien and outside my experience, but on the other hand a most intense ...*déjà vu* ... as if I knew that dark-skinned man who had been waiting for me for five thousand years' (ibid.). Here is the pivotal example of Jung holding simultaneously together both sides of his paradoxical experience of the primitive: utterly alien and long awaited. A new attitude transcends the conflict of negative and positive. If we were speaking in Jung's 'scientific' language of translating psychic image into clinical concept, we may say this was conscious recognition of Self linking with ego and ego linking with Self, both ways—a revelation.

Jung thought he went to Africa to investigate the primitive life outside of Europe and his civilized identity. He discovered instead Africa investigating him, bringing to awareness primitive parts of him. This sets in larger context racist remarks and reductionism of Blacks to the primitive. Instead of an objective study of the primitive in Africa, Jung was led to a subjective study of missing primitive parts of himself and to more positive parts of blackness in himself than he imagined (ibid., pp. 244–45, 273). Here are acknowledged black parts central to him: the small brown man helping him murder Siegfried; the murderous combat with the Arab who becomes a boy who must learn the book; the tall spear-man with whom he links after five thousand years of waiting to do so. These are figures Jung deeply feels and honors.

These black men give Jung firsthand experiences of their lives, linking him to psyche's taproot. In this meeting with the spear-man, there followed Jung's experience in Nairobi with dazzling light and the vast plains of the Athi game preserve, trod by thousands of animals. He saw himself seeing the objectivity of creation before him. His myth by which he was to live was revealed to him: 'There the cosmic meaning of consciousness became overwhelmingly clear to me ... . Man (sic) is the second creator of the world, who alone has given to the world its objective existence' (Jung 1961/1963, pp. 255–56).

Training students

To reckon with Jung's paradoxical relation to the primitive provides force in teaching. To touch upon a racist text or upon the notion of the Black as emissary of the Self in Jung's experience is to evoke still current ambivalences to blackness in the emotional field of learning in the class. Candidates and teachers may be shocked to feel the primitive opened up right then in themselves, with all its brutality and cover-ups of sentimentality. To perceive collusion with a white collective equation that erases the *isness* of Blacks in all their diversity arouses horror and shame amidst the false symbolization of Blacks as repudiated parts of white selves. Equally strong is the opposition between racist remarks and Jung's honoring blackness in himself that has been waiting for him for five thousand years. To see repudiated parts—the rejected, lowly, feared, spit upon—as the carrier of engagement with the center evokes wonder, honor ... feelings too deep for words.

The ever-present disparity of equality between teacher and student decreases as class members realize this applies to all of us facing primitive in us with the tide of remorse for harm done, of fierce aggressiveness, of flooding insight like the dazzling light of creation, of darkness so deep it changes the mode of communication to reach it and speak together of it. Curiosity rises: What are the archetypal images of countries in Africa? In the Caribbean? What are the archetypes of slavery, of overcoming it? What images fuel the diversity within Black culture? How to process the strength in Billie Holiday singing 'Strange Fruit', of the fortitude of Black thinkers, of the color in the paintings of Romare Bearden and Alma Woodsey Thomas?

Will this change anything? Yes, by increments. If we touch the primitive in our teaching and learning, it will touch us. We can tolerate not knowing and finding different ways to communicate what we and it fashions between us.

Note

1   I cite 'Negroes' when Jung does; otherwise, I cite 'Blacks' to refer to this ethnic group.

References

Brewster, F. (2013). 'Wheel of fire: the African American dreamer and cultural unconsciousness'. *Jung Journal: Culture and Psyche*, 7, 1, 70–87.

Bright. G. (2021). 'Book review of *The Black Books 1913–1932: Notebooks of Transformation*'. *Journal of Analytical Psychology*, 66, 3, 763–775.

Jung, C.G. (1913–1932/2020). *The Black Books: Notebooks of Transformation*, ed. S. Shamdasani. New York and London: W.W. Norton.

Jung, C.G. (1921). *Psychological Types. Collected Works (CW) 6*.

Jung, C.G. (1930/1939/1976). 'A radio talk in Munich'. *CW 18*.

Jung, C.G. (1931/1964). 'The archaic man'. *CW 10*.

Jung, C.G. (1932/1997). 'Spring Term, Lecture Two' (11 May 1932). *Visions, Vol. 2: Notes of the Seminar Given in 1930–1934 by C. G. Jung*. Claire Douglas, ed. Princeton: Princeton University Press.

Jung, C.G. (1935/1939/1976). 'Tavistock lectures, II'. *CW 18*.

Jung, C.G. (1939/1976). 'The symbolic life'. *CW 18*.

Jung, C.G. (1961/1963). *Memories, Dreams, Reflections*, rec. & ed.A. Jaffe, trans. R. & C. Winston. New York: Pantheon Books of Random House.

Jung, C.G. (2009). *The Red Book: Liber Novus*, ed. S. Shamdasani. New York: W.W. Norton.

Morgan, H. (2021). *The Work of Whiteness: A Psychoanalytic Perspective*. New York and Oxford: Routledge.

Skerritt, H.F., ed. (2016). *Marking the Infinite Contemporary Women Artists from Aboriginal Australia*. London, New York: Nevada Museum of Art, Delmonico Books, Prestel.

Ulanov, A.B. (2015). 'Jung, psychic reality, and God'. *Jung and the Academy and Beyond The Fordham Lectures 100 Years Later*, eds. M. Mattson, F. Wertz, H. Fogarty, M. Klenck & B. Zabriskie (pp. 165–187). New Orleans, LA: Spring Journal Books.

Ulanov, A.B. (2020). *Knots and Their Untying: Essays on Psychological Dilemmas*. Einsiedeln: Daimon Verlag.

Ulanov, A.B. (2022). *Back to Basics*. Einsiedeln, Switzerland: Daimon Verlag.

Chapter 3

The Smoking Mirror

An archetypal perspective on the color black

Deborah Fausch

In *The Fire Next Time*, the writer and cultural activist James Baldwin observes:

> [T]he racial tensions that menace Americans today have little to do with real antipathy—on the contrary, indeed—and are involved only symbolically with color. Those tensions are rooted in the very same depths as those from which love springs, or murder. The white man's unadmitted—and apparently, to him, unspeakable—private fears and longings are projected onto the Negro. The only way he can be released from the Negro's tyrannical power over him is to consent, in effect, to become black himself, to become part of that suffering and dancing country that he now watches wistfully from the heights of his lonely power.
>
> (Baldwin 1962/1998, pp. 341–42)

As I write (14 May 2022), 13 persons have been shot and ten killed in a grocery store in Buffalo, New York. The reason for targeting them was that they were Black. Celebrating the horrifying lunacy of Great Replacement Theory on social media, the 18-year-old gunman posted that by their very existence, Black Americans threaten to replace white Americans—a reversal of the truth that to have dark skin in America is to risk death daily.[1] As Ibram X. Kendi declared, 'Black people are facing the double terror of racist policy and racist violence' (Kendi 2022, n.p.).

Beyond the projection of disavowed complexes onto Black persons; beyond the deliberate demonization of "others" by politicians and news commentators that may have led the gunman to see massacre as the solution to his fears; beyond the instability and isolation experienced by many young males; beyond even the history of hatred, rejection, oppression and violence toward persons of African heritage in the United States, part of its very founding as a nation; beyond these, what else is operating underneath the forces in such furious play? Our cultural constructs make use of archetypal images linked to deep patterns in the human psyche. These patterns add additional intensity to our interactions, fueling the dynamics of othering, oppression, and violence. Amplifying the archetypal qualities of black allows

DOI: 10.4324/9781003311447-4

us to distinguish cultural complexes from archetypal appearances, and conversely to see the weight of the archetypal in the cultural.

In this exploration of the historical, cultural, and archetypal resonances of the color black, I have taken heart from Baldwin's deep understanding of the inner psychology of racism. Baldwin saw clearly that the cure for racism lies in our collective self-examination. As he eloquently articulates, the topic of black—and its opposite color white—can be addressed only from the most personal and individual of standpoints:

> What you say about somebody else, anybody else, reveals *you*. What I think of you as being is dictated by my own necessity, my own psychology, my own fears and desires. I'm not describing you when I talk about you; I'm describing me.
>
> (Baldwin & Luster 1964, n.p.)

Baldwin insisted on honest, loving dialogue as interdependent partners in creating an American identity of freedom, unity and equality for us all.

This chapter consists of three sections. The first is a short resume of the color complex of blackness in the United States and its roots in English natural philosophy and history. Black, in this section, is flat black, embodying opposition, projection, oppression, trauma. The second opens the historical view of black to its archetypal base, showing that black contains within itself the opposites that are characteristic of an archetypal structure. This section also demonstrates the richness of the color in various symbolic systems. The final section explores the relationship between color as culturally defined and color as an archetypal structure, and explores the question whether an enriched idea of blackness can help to heal the racial trauma that persists in the United States.

Cultural complexes

Although America's history is tainted by racism directed against persons whose skin color is designated as "yellow", "red", and "brown" as well as black, the color black functions as a condensation and symbol of the racial problems that haunt American culture and the American psyche, containing within its emblematic imagery the conflicting values and experiences of over 400 years of trauma (Menakem 2017). It is an image of what Thomas Singer and Samuel L. Kimbles (2004) term a 'cultural complex'.

Carl Jung described complexes as collections of feelings, ideas, and experiences that often originate in a traumatic experience, 'an emotional shock ... that splits off a bit of the psyche' (Jung 1960, para. 204). This original experience and affect collect related ideas and feelings around themselves. The complex then behaves like a 'splinter psyche', an organized, unconscious center that can take over an individual's thoughts, feelings, and behavior, expressing itself in strong emotions and repetitive behaviors that tend to reinforce the complex's view of the world. Thus, complexes structure the individual's experiences and perceptions of self and others. Paola Palmiotto notes that 'feeling-toned complexes, bypassing the cortex, activate the limbic system in a state of alarm. Often this reaction is exaggerated with respect to the external stimuli, a wrong perception of the danger that is internalized in the person' (Palmiotto 2016).

Cultures have some of the same structures as individuals. Like individual egos, they are consciously structured around commonly-agreed-upon sets of ideas and values. As an individual's unconscious shadow contains those elements of the person's personality that are intolerable to the conscious ego and are projected onto others, so also the rejected qualities of cultural values are projected onto those designated as "other". '[T]he group ego or the individual ego of a group member becomes identified with one part of a cultural complex, while the other part is projected onto the suitable hook of another group or one of its members' (Singer & Kimbles 2004, p. 6). This basic projective mechanism substantiates Baldwin's assertion that in talking about the other, we talk about ourselves.

Kimbles (2014) stresses that cultural complexes are connected to archetypal structures of sameness and difference; these function to simplify the inherently ambiguous realities of group identity by means of projection and introjection. The push toward simplified, oppositional ways of experiencing reality is evidence of a bipolar archetypal underpinning that contributes to "black-and-white" thinking, as the shadow side of the complex is disavowed by those in its grip and projected onto others. '[L]ike individual complexes, cultural complexes tend to be repetitive, autonomous, resist consciousness, and collect experience that confirms their historical point of view' (Singer & Kimbles 2004, p. 6). This mechanism is underscored by Audrey and Brian Smedley:

> We think we "see" race when we encounter certain physical differences among people such as skin color, eye shape, and hair texture. What we actually "see" … are the learned social meanings, the stereotypes, that have been linked to those physical features by the ideology of race and the historical legacy it has left us.
> (Audrey & Brian Smedley 2012; in Isabel Wilkerson 2020, p. 67)

Thus we see through the lenses of our cultural complexes.

Cultural complexes operate at the level of inner image and fantasy. Their intergenerational images give ghostly substance to narratives that invisibly hold sway in the psyches of present-day individuals. Kimbles (2014, p. 29) calls these narratives 'phantoms'—'absent subjectivities [that] haunt the present'—embodied in unconsciously held attitudes, beliefs, and ways of being that refer to past traumas without specific memory of them.

America's color complex

In *Caste: The Origins of Our Discontents*, Isabel Wilkerson states: 'Color is a fact. Race is a social construct' (Wilkerson 2020, p. 66). Both intellectually and culturally, color functions as a means for marking differences, separating the world's 'blooming, buzzing confusion' into this and not-this—a necessary simplification of the endless variety of things into oppositional categories.[2] As the historian of color Michel Pastoureau observes, 'in every society color's first function is to classify, mark, proclaim, combine, or contrast' (Michel Pastoureau 2009, p. 16). Essayist William Gass concurs:

> Colors ... allow us to discriminate among otherwise identical things (gold and green racing cars, football teams, jelly beans, red- brown- blond- and black-haired girls); however, our eye is always at the edge, establishing boundaries, making claims, so that colors principally enable us to discern shapes and define relations, and it certainly appears that patterns and paths—first, last, and in between—are what we want and what we remember: useful contraptions, useful controls, and useful connections.
> (Gass 1976/2014, pp. 61–62)

This use of color for discriminating amongst 'otherwise identical things' has furnished the basis for distinctions among persons from very early times. In ancient Hindu society, the four *varnas* were *Brahmin* (priests), *Kshatriya* (warriors), *Vaishya* (merchants), and *Shudra* (laborers), along with the excluded *avarna*, the Untouchables or *Dalits*. These distinctions were color-based. In the *Rig Veda, varna* means 'colour, outward appearance, exterior, form, figure or shape'. In the *Mahabharata*, the word (signifying 'color, tint, dye or pigment') refers to 'colour, race, tribe, species, kind, sort, nature, character, quality, property' (Monier-Williams 1899/2005, p. 924). The worst fate was to be *avarna*, without color—not to have any place in the social schema. Siimilarly, in the West until late medieval times, the three traditional classes of human beings were color-coded as white (priests), red (warriors) and black (laborers). This organization has Indo-European roots (Dumézil 1954, pp. 45–61) and can be seen as far back as ancient Rome, where different segments of society wore clothing based on their occupations: purple for the emperor, white for priests, red for warriors, and a dull black for craftsmen and artisans (Warburton 2014, p. 6).

In contrast to the relatively lower social ranking of laborers, craftsmen and artisans, for some cultures—the inhabitants of Taquile and Uros in Peru, the nobility of early modern Europe, and the formally dressed in contemporary society (Houck-Loomis 2022; Pastoureau 2009)—the wearing of black has served as a marker of high status. However, when such cultural constructs are allied to power and scapegoating, they become oppressive and even lethal. Colorism, a social hierarchy based on skin color, is indeed a cultural complex that has deep roots in all our souls. As Kathy Russell-Cole, Midge Wilson, and Ronald E. Hall describe in *The Color Complex* (2013), the construal of lighter skin as higher in status than darker skin has been found in most cultures across history and geography, from India to Asia to Latin America to Europe. Originating in the stratification of early agricultural societies, it differentiated those who labored outside from those with more wealth and status whose indoor work involved managing laborers. Often, men were seen as "properly" darker than women (Russell-Cole et al. 2013, pp. 85–86). Ancient Egyptian wall paintings depict male figures with red skin and female figures with white skin; likewise, in ancient Greek and Roman art, female figures were often depicted with light-colored skin as befitted their indoor lives, whereas male figures, who were meant to be outside working or fighting, had dark-colored skin (McDaniel 2020). Especially in patriarchies, upper-class women were typically sequestered in the home. The lighter the skin, the less time the woman had spent outdoors, and the higher status she therefore possessed (Russell-Cole et al. 2013, pp. 26–30). This association with leisure and light skin also reigned in colonial Barbados and South Carolina, where, according to the American historian Winthrop D. Jordan, white upper-class women were positioned as "upholding the race". They were expected to be remotely, politely asexual and without any hint of tanned skin, thus unassociated with outdoor work (Jordan 1968, p. 148). Only in the 20th century did darker skin become a status marker for persons of northern European ancestry, when a tan indicated that one had the leisure for outdoor sport.

Within the gradation from dark to light, a common cultural structure is a three-tier distinction of dark, medium-tone, and light skin, more properly termed 'color discrimination' than racial discrimination (Russell-Cole et al. 2013, p. 32). But in the color hierarchy of the United States, the history of slavery caused this gradation to be simplified into a "black/white" caste system in which those of non-European ancestry, whether "brown", "red", or "yellow", were classed as "not white".

As Wilkerson describes, Colorism is one part of the larger structure of caste, in which the phenomenology of skin color and the social construction of "race" are overlaid by the ideology of caste. Caste systems fix and harden gradations into divisions through what Wilkerson terms its 'eight pillars': 1) the assertion of divine will and natural law in the division of "races"; 2) the enforcement of the heritability of caste position; 3) the prohibition of marriage between or among castes; 4) schemas of purity and pollution; 5) hierarchies of occupations; 6) dehumanization of, and stigma attached to, those of lower caste; 7) use of terror and cruelty to keep lower caste persons in their assigned place; and 8) assertions of inherent superiority and inferiority. These social strictures are rooted in archetypal structures that find expression in dominance and scapegoating.

Cultures are constituted as much by what they exclude as by what they include, and part of the attraction of caste systems (for those identified as being of higher caste) is archetypal in nature: the division into bipolar opposites and the appeal to fixed categories are felt to be undergirded by divine and natural law. But in *Purity and Danger* (1966/2002), anthropologist Mary Douglas emphasizes the human origins of these categories. Douglas disagrees with John Locke's perspective that our minds, or our cultures, are blank slates; rather, she asserts that 'conception determines perception' in a reciprocal relationship between our categories and our experience:

> [W]hatever we perceive is organised into patterns for which we, the perceivers, are largely responsible. Perceiving is not a matter of passively allowing an organ—say of sight or hearing—to receive a ready-made impression from without, like a palette receiving a spot of paint. Recognising and remembering are not matters of stirring up old images of past impressions. It is generally agreed that all our impressions are schematically determined from the start.
>
> (Douglas 1966/2002, p. 45)

Douglas shows that the need to 'impose system on an unruly experience' (1966/2002, p. 5) causes cultures to slot phenomena into fixed, opposing classes by means of proscriptions and taboos. As exemplified in the dietary exclusion laws found in *Leviticus*, these taboos work to create categories and boundaries by projecting onto scapegoats what is construed as "not us".[3] Partly because color itself is archetypal, differences in skin color lend themselves to taboos and scapegoating, the building blocks of caste systems. The history of the color black in the West, and its use to label, stereotype, and discriminate against people with darker skin, shows evidence of this archetypal undergirding.

Blackness in English and American culture and history

In *Stamped from the Beginning* (2016), Ibram X. Kendi relates the history of the deployment of racial constructs already embedded in European thought to ensure continued access to enslaved labor in the United States. Kendi asserts that the need for power over a captive labor force preceded and prescribed determinations of "race". Beginning in the early 17th century, a series of legal decisions were formulated to progressively define Africans and persons of African descent as essentially other than European, and thus not entitled to equal rights. Legislation that defined a person's "race" by his/her mother's identity recast centuries of British law in terms that fostered inherited slavery. Anthropologist Ashley Montagu (1945) writes, 'The idea of race, was, in fact, the deliberate creation of an exploiting class seeking to maintain and defend its privileges against what was profitably regarded as an inferior caste' (Wilkerson 2020, pp. 65–66).

To understand the history of the "color bar" in America, Winthrop Jordan believes we must start with the attitudes predominant in the Protestant world of the English colonists. Jordan defines "attitudes" in terms that suggest the psychic mechanisms of cultural complexes:

> I have taken "attitudes" to be discrete entities susceptible of historical analysis. This term ... suggests thoughts and feelings (as opposed to actions) directed toward some specific object (as opposed to generalized faiths and beliefs). At the same time it suggests a wide range in consciousness, intensity, and saliency in the response to the object ... . [Attitudes exist] not only at various levels of intensity but at various levels of consciousness and unconsciousness; ... there is no clear dividing line between "thought" and "feeling," between conscious and unconscious mental processes.
>
> (Jordan 1968, p. xxvii)

Teasing out the attitudes that fostered the persistence of slavery and segregation in America, Jordan describes the amazement of the British at the darkness of the West African and Congolese persons they encountered in the mid-1500s. Their perception of Africans as different from themselves was mapped both onto their prior understanding of the symbolic qualities of black and white and onto an inherited tradition of mythical beasts and half-human creatures located in the southern regions of the world. As Jordan notes:

> No other color except white conveyed so much emotional impact [as black]. As described by the *Oxford English Dictionary*, the meaning of black before the sixteenth century included, 'Deeply stained with dirt; soiled, dirty, foul ... . Having dark or deadly purposes, malignant; pertaining to or involving death, deadly; baneful, disastrous, sinister ... . Foul, iniquitous, atrocious, horrible, wicked ... . Indicating disgrace, censure, liability to punishment, etc.' Black was an emotionally partisan color, the handmaid and symbol of baseness and evil, a sign of danger and repulsion. Embedded in the concept of blackness was its direct opposite—whiteness. No other colors so clearly implied opposition, "beinge coloures utterlye contrary"; no others were so frequently used to denote polarization.
>
> (Jordan 1968, p. 7)

At the time of its first contact with black Africans, English society was undergoing enormous shifts from a highly structured medieval society to a modern one, at once more open and unstructured outwardly and more introspective inwardly. Added to this upheaval and uncertainty was the colonists' need to create a new identity for themselves in the New World. In this search for identity, the traditional opposition of black and white was powerfully influential. The division of humans by color construed Africans and persons of African ancestry as irreducibly different from English persons, and the dichotomous color code provided a convenient rationale for projection of what could not be countenanced as "mine":

Many pious Englishmen, not all of them "Puritans," came to approach life as if conducting an examination and to approach Scripture as if peering in a mirror. As a result, their inner energies were brought unusually close to the surface, more frequently into the almost rational world of legend, myth, and literature ... . Given this charged atmosphere of (self-) discovery, it is scarcely surprising that Englishmen should have used peoples overseas as social mirrors and that they were especially inclined to discover attributes in savages which they found first but could not speak of in themselves.

(Jordan 1968, pp. 39–40)

Jordan claims that: '[r]ather than slavery causing "prejudice", or vice versa, they seem rather to have generated each other ... . Slavery and "prejudice" may have been equally cause and effect, continuously reacting upon each other' (Jordan 1968, p. 80). His conclusion is supported by Douglas's description of the reciprocal relationship between conception and perception and explains how the 'social mirroring' of white by black became key to the development of an American identity.

In these early associations to black and white, color was not merely a secondary quality of objects but was inextricably interwoven with the materiality and spirituality of things. As an archetypal structure, it tied together all levels of being in a satisfying, signifying whole, and was thus also an index of moral qualities. But in the 17th century, Robert Boyle and Isaac Newton replaced the traditional Aristotelian color theory inherited via religion and alchemy with new theories based on experimentation. As James Hillman notes:

The new optics embodied other fantasies about the sensate world, displacing the alchemical importance of colors as revelations of essential nature with inherent psychological properties, the very manifestations of the divine, God's rainbow, guaranteeing His presence in the raiment of things. Alchemical colors are in the world, of the world, and tell about the world. After Newton and Locke (1690, first draft 1672), colors are refractions of light, neither a sign of mystery nor an essential virtue, rather a secondary effect produced in the human understanding by abstract laws.

(Hillman 1986, p. 44)

Primarily concerned with reflection and absorption of light, and its wave-lengths, Boyle's and Newton's treatises still carried some of the earlier archetypal overtones. Directing a beam of sunlight through a pyramid, Newton (1672) discerned seven colors in the rainbow, to harmonize with the archetypal resonances of the number seven and the seven tones of the Western musical scale. Boyle's treatise (1664) came to cultural as well as scientific conclusions. He theorized that whiteness was created by smooth, reflective surfaces, while blackness was created by rough, absorptive surfaces. The great majority of the essay was devoted to experiments proving these hypotheses, but in 'Experiment XI', Boyle considered the possible reasons that Africans' "black" skin varied from what he considered to be normative "white" skin color.[4] He concluded that dark skin is due neither to greater sun exposure nor to the curse of Noah on his son 'Cham' (Ham), two explanations popular at the time. Boyle noted that, as evidenced by dissection, skin color is literally skin-deep, and there is no essential difference between humans of varying skin tones:

> Nor is it evident that Blackness is a Curse, for Navigators tell us of Black Nations, who think so much otherwise of their own condition, that they paint the Devil White. Nor is Blackness inconsistent with Beauty, which even to our European Eyes consists not so much in Colour, as an Advantageous Stature, a Comely Symmetry of the parts of the Body, and Good Features in the Face. So that I see not why Blackness should be thought such a Curse to the Negroe.
>
> (Boyle 1664, p. 160)

Boyle's even-handed assessment is remarkable for his times, but why did he feel the need, in a treatise almost entirely devoted to the corpuscular nature of surfaces as the causes of colored light, to insert a discussion of skin color? A member of the Council on Foreign Plantations, Boyle was charged with overseeing the Crown's colonial properties. His conclusion that we are all equal did not prevent him from assuring slave owners in Barbados and the continental colonies that, their slaves need not be freed, although they ought to be converted to Christianity (Kendi 2016, p. 45).

Even more influential than Boyle's and Newton's investigations was John Locke's *An Essay in Human Understanding* (1690/2019), a cornerstone of the natural rights philosophy that undergirded the new American Republic. Like Boyle, Locke was involved in administering the British colonial enterprise. As the secretary to the Lords Proprietors of the Carolina colonies, he composed the *Fundamental Constitution of the Carolinas*, which gave plantation owners absolute power over the enslaved.

Perhaps this role motivated his interest in defining the essential characteristics of human beings. Although he devotes several pages of his treatise to the entertaining story of a talking parrot, Locke argues that we relate most strongly to 'creatures of our own shape or make', regardless of their ability to reason (Locke 1690/2019, Book III, Chapter III, p. 416). In line with contemporary beliefs in appearance as a reliable key to inner nature, he emphasizes that it is the visual qualities of humanness that matter. However, Locke also examines the inductive reasoning of an English child, who generalizes erroneously from visual experience to a category. The example makes the point that those who deny black persons full humanity employ flawed logic:

> First, a child having framed the idea of a man, it is probable that his idea is just like that picture which the painter makes of the visible appearances joined together; and such a complication of ideas together in his understanding makes up the single complex idea which he calls man, whereof white or flesh-colour in England being one, the child can demonstrate to you that a negro is not a man, because white colour was one of the constant simple ideas of the complex idea he calls man; and therefore he can demonstrate, by the principle, It is impossible for the same thing to be and not to be, that a negro is not a man; the foundation of his certainty being not that universal proposition, which perhaps he never heard nor thought of, but the clear, distinct perception he hath of his own simple ideas of black and white, which he cannot be persuaded to take, nor can ever mistake one for another, whether he knows that maxim or no.
>
> (Locke 1690/2019, Book IV, Chapter VII, p. 627)

Locke's musings are of particular importance because of his influence on the philosophy that undergirded the formation of the Constitution of the United States. By 1680, "English", "Christian", "white", and "free" had become synonymous with correct behavior and attitudes as well as full citizenship, while Africans were construed as strange, "heathen", black, and therefore suitable for enslavement (Jordan 1968, pp. 94–97). A nation founded on the philosophy of natural human rights, however, could not logically validate slavery, and Jordan describes the Framers' struggles to square the belief in the equality of all humankind with the perceived need for slavery in the "lower South" of South Carolina and Georgia. Contemporary outcry acknowledging the essential equality of the enslaved pressed for manumission, but the abolitionist movement foundered on the twin need for labor in Southern states and a pervasive sense of otherness that focused on the physical traits, especially skin color, of Africans and their enslaved descendents. By the early 1800s, this sense of otherness had hardened into a determination, shared by many including Thomas Jefferson, that there should be no "racial mixing". This conviction stemmed from what we would term an unconscious complex that projected sexuality, aggression, mental inferiority, and sheer animal-ness onto Africans and their colonized descendants. Simultaneously, however, Jefferson considered slavery an unmitigated evil that must be abolished for the new nation to achieve its ideals. The longer the contradiction between the nation's ideals and the reality of slavery persisted, the greater the need for these projections—and the more the sense of inferior otherness was concretized. Thus, unequal otherness was critical to the construction of America's identity, and the new nation seemed resolved that black serve as a mirror in which white might see and know itself.

Archetypal black

As is evident in the early modern English conceptions of black and white, the need for clear-cut opposites and hierarchy is inherent in the archetypal qualities of the color white, which contains ideas of purity, innocence, transcendence, spiritualization, and superiority, an "us" that requires a "them" for its foil. Hillman (1986) describes this characteristic as 'the delusional snow job of white supremacy which forces distinctions into oppositions, splitting white and black'. He continues:

> Differences neither compete, contradict nor oppose. To be as different as night and day does not require an opposition of night and day … . [But] it is archetypally given with whiteness to imagine in oppositions. To say it again: *the supremacy of white depends on oppositional imagining* [italics in original]. …
> [Thus] we now experience projection to be the very essence of our high civilization.
>
> (Hillman 1986, pp. 39, 41, 47)

In projection, the division into opposites intersects with the archetypal structure of hierarchy. White/black maps onto good/evil, layering a potentially harmful configuration of hierarchical value onto that of opposition. Such hierarchizing lends itself to debasing, and on a cultural level projection and projective identification occur as the demonization of one group by another.

Archetypally as well as culturally, white demands to be mirrored in black, defining itself by what it is not. Black, however, does not need to be mirrored in this way. Partaking of a *coincidentia oppositorum*—both fruitful and deadly, good and evil, madonna and devil—it contains within itself the essential polarity of an archetypal structure. Black has a self-sufficiency that does not need to be constituted in relationship to white and has the capacity to absorb and reflect back all that it encounters.

In *Black: The History of a Color* (2009), Pastoureau insists that '[i]t is the society that "makes" the color, that gives it its definitions and meanings, that constructs its codes and values, that organizes its customs and determines its stakes' (Pastoureau 2009, pp. 16–17). Yet he admits that there are archetypal aspects to color:

> I am forced to acknowledge that a few chromatic referents are encountered in almost every society. They are not numerous: fire and blood for red; vegetation for green; light for white; night for black—an ambivalent, even ambiguous night, yes, but always, everywhere, more disturbing or destructive than fertile or comforting.
>
> (Pastoureau 2009, p. 24)

Pastoureau's preliminary discussion of black demonstrates its ambivalent, ambiguous, double-valued structure, grounded in resonances of humanity's earliest, archetypal experiences and ideas: the darkness of the cosmos before creation occurs; our fear of darkness before the discovery of fire; and conversely, the fertility of black soil and dark rain clouds. This fertile aspect is embodied in black deities, including earth goddesses Demeter, Ceres, Hecate, Isis, Kali, and the Black Madonna. It is also personified in gods such as Vishnu, 'black as a full rain cloud'; blue-black skinned Krishna of compassionate, loving, protective nature, whose name means "black", "dark", or "dark blue"; underworld Osiris, god of death and rebirth, colored black and green. Egypt's nurturing black silt, brought down by the Nile in its annual flood, is the source of its name *Kemet*, the black land. Fertile, fecund black is also associated with underground locations where gods are born and where humans have worshipped and undergone rites of passage (Pastoureau 2009, pp. 21–24).

We can distinguish several clusters of meaning for this powerful color. First, it is related to the primordial, that which existed before the beginning—the void, the nonmanifest—or the beginning itself:

> Black, in fairly generalized terms, seems to represent the initial, germinal stage of all processes, as it does in alchemy ... . Black crows, black doves and black flames figure in a great many legends. They are all symbols closely related to the primal (black, occult or unconscious) wisdom which stems from the Hidden Source ... . [T]he profoundest meaning of black is occultation and germination in darkness.
>
> (Circlot 1962/1971, p. 57)

From this absolute *increatum* comes the association of unchanging eternal presence and constancy, before and beyond the particulars of the created world (de Vries & de Vries 1974/2004, p. 67). For example, the Masai creation myth features two gods. The Red God, Naiterukop, is the creator of the earth, but the Black God—the God of the Dead, the Night, and the Beyond—is outside of creation, and therefore greater than the Red God. Death is life in the Beyond, where the dead continue living 'in the preconscious totality' (von Franz 1972/1995, pp. 103, 115–16).

In ancient Greek cosmology, black is likewise there from the beginning. Nyx (Night) stands at the start of creation; Hesiod called her 'mother of the gods'. The daughter of Chaos, the primordial void, Nyx brings forth Uranus and Gaia, Heaven and Earth. By day, she resides in a dark cave in the West; by night, she rides across the sky clothed in black and pulled by four black horses. Her children include the positive deities of Sleep and Dreams, as well as the negative ones of Anguish, Secrets, Discord, Distress, Old Age, Misfortune, and Death, and perhaps the Furies, the Fates, and

Nemesis (Pastoureau 2009, p. 21). Night's darkness contains the antipodes of human life, daylight's promise and the day's end.

The Zuni creation myth begins with the creator god Awonawilona alone in the 'black darkness and void'. Awonawilona conceives a thought, which takes shape and 'steps out into the void', turning into 'nebulae of growth and mist, full of power of growth'. Then Awonawilona changes himself into the sun, 'who is our father and who enlightens everything and fills everything with light', and the nebulae sink down and become the sea (von Franz 1972/1995, p. 203). Marie-Louise Von Franz states that the sun is a symbol of consciousness and the sea symbolizes the unconscious, and she notes that the opposites of consciousness and unconsciousness come into being simultaneously. Before this split, there is only the all-embracing totality that contains everything. Chaotic and pregnant, blackness is the state before differentiation.

Once differentiation occurs, it is in the archetypal nature of color itself that black typically occurs in opposition to another color. White and black together symbolize 'the ceaseless alternations of life/death, light/darkness and appearance/disappearance which make possible the continued existence of phenomena' (Circlot 1962/1971, p. 59). In one Chinese creation story, the universe begins as structureless chaos within which there eventually coalesces a black egg containing a huge hairy giant, Pangu. Pangu sleeps in the egg for more than 18,000 years, during which the universe is perfectly balanced, with equal amounts of darkness (*yin*) and light (*yang*). When Pangu escapes the egg, breaking the force that has kept the universe in equilibrium, the top half of the egg shell, representing *yang*, turns into the sky. The bottom half, representing *yin*, becomes the earth. All earth's creatures are created of Pangu's body (Dehai et al. 2018, p. 11). The Judeo-Christian creation myth tells a similar story. The original potential space—'darkness on the face of the deep'—is followed by God's declaration: 'Let there be light' (*Genesis* 1: 2–3). After the first, eternal moment of formless void, light comes and darkness begins to participate in opposition.

Representing the '"descent into hell", a recapitulation of (or an atonement for) all the preceding phases' (Circlot 1962/1971, p. 58), black also becomes the preliminary stage of the next thing. Jean Cooper (1978) also connects black to movement in time—'hard, pitiless and irrational'—by means of Saturn (C(h)ronos) and Kali. The dark aspect of the Great Mother, black-skinned Kali's name is related to *Kala*, "time" (Cooper 1978, p. 39). This time is cyclical, as Hillman describes in his essay on alchemical black:

Alchemical psychology teaches us to read as accomplishments the fruitlessly bitter and dry periods [of the *nigredo*, the period of black depression], the melancholies that seem never to end, the wounds that do not heal, the grinding sadistic mortifications of shame and the putrefactions of love and friendships. These are beginnings because they are

endings, dissolutions, deconstructions. But they are not the beginning, as a one-time-only occurrence. ... [T]he alchemical process ... is an *iteratio*.
(Hillman 1997/2010, loc. 1735–38)

Black grounds humans not only in time but in space. The world's four quarters and the vertical world axis are traditionally signified by colors, and the correspondences of all levels of existence are held together by means of these colors. In these orientation systems, black is commonly associated with the North, from which comes rain and winter; thus Finno-Ugrics sacrificed black animals to water deities, and in China, the color has influence over the bladder and kidneys. In ancient Egypt, where it was connected to the direction of the setting sun (thematic of death and rebirth), black was associated with the gall bladder and liver (Jobes 1962, p. 221).

Black and white, good and bad

Black as night, the black of the unknown, of dark caves and thick woods— things are black when we can't envision, can't understand, are unaware, when we "black out", go unconscious, have blackouts, forgetting whole segments of time. Black tends to carry the negative, both in the sense of the unconscious, the unexpressed, and the hidden, and in the sense of negative mood and value. From early on, black represented death. In ancient Egypt, death was associated with Thoth, the conductor of souls, whose head is a black Ibis. Anubis, god of the underworld, took the form of a black jackal who protected the dead. For the Greeks the realm of death was ruled by Erebus, son of Chaos and brother of Night. It included Tartarus, the deepest, darkest region of hell, where Hades sat on an ebony throne. By Roman times, *Nox* (night) was noxious, black meant dirty, gloomy, malevolent, and deathly, and dark colors were worn for mourning (Pastoureau 2009, p. 35).

Psychologically, black is the color of depressed mood, as heavy as lead, the metal associated with the black, malefic god Saturn (de Vries & de Vries, 1974/2004, p. 67). In the Western traditional fourfold relationship of colors, humors, and temperaments, black represented the melancholic temperament, characterized by an excess of black bile (μέλαινα χολή; *melaina chole*), which caused the darkening of blood and depression. Thus, melancholic persons were depicted with black faces. Likewise, in Hinduism's three-part division of energies and ways of being, black is the color of *tamas* (darkness), a state characterized by chaos, imbalance, disorder, chaos, anxiety, impurity, destruction, delusion, apathy, and inertia. *Rajas* (activity and passion) is colored red. *Sattva* (knowledge, love, and harmony) is white.

In Europe, black has often occurred in opposition to another color. This opposition is first found in Pythagoras's 'Table of Opposites', which Aristotle recorded as ten bipolar pairs, including dark/light, right/left, male/female, one/many, and good/evil (Aristotle 2016, *Metaphysics* A 5 986a22–b2, pp. 12–13).

This table represented symbolic classifications with socioethical implications, 'according to which the presence of a principle on one column of the table will carry with it another principle within the same column' (Goldin 2015, p. 172). Thus in Pythagoras's prescientific world view, things were held together as a mutually entailed whole, characterized by oppositional forces.

In ancient, medieval and early Renaissance alchemy, however, and throughout Africa, the most salient combination of colors is not the opposition of black and white, but the traditional primary-color triad of black-white-red (McNatt 2007). The world is divided into three active principles embodied in these three colors as archetypal processes. One of the best-documented examples of this schema is found in the Ndembu, a Zambian group studied by the anthropologist Victor Turner. The Ndembu conceive of the three principles of black, white, and red as 'rivers of power' flowing from the divine source. The three colors embody experiences, powers, and social relationships, thus tying the entire world together into a meaningful set of actions, relationships, objects, and ideas. Turner ties the three colors to human biology and affective experience and makes the point that the colors are linked to underlying archetypal structures: '[t]hough immanent in man's [sic] body, they appear to transcend his [sic] consciousness. ... [T]he forces and symbols for them are biologically, psychologically, and logically prior to social classifications by moieties, clans, sex totems and all the rest of experience' (Turner 1967, p. 90).

Like the Ndembu culture, the Arab and Western practice of alchemy was organized around the three primary colors of black, white, and red. The Great Work of transformation, from leaden base materials to noble gold, from ignorant initiate to possessor of the Philosopher's Stone of the Wise, consisted of a series of stages colored black, white, and red, each of which embodied both processes and states of being. Like the rituals of the Ndembu, the alchemical processes of *calcinatio, solutio, coagulatio, sublimatio, mortificatio* or *putrefactio, separatio* and *coniunctio* operated in a world where color signified the essential nature of the thing it tinged, and a change in color meant a change in substance. And in these colors, matter and spirit, physical and symbolic, were also inextricably intertwined.

Jung sees the alchemical process as an image of the process of individuation, the life-long process of becoming oneself. By faithfully following the developments in the retort from *nigredo* to *albedo* to *rubedo*, the alchemist could transform him- or herself from ignorance to wisdom, unconsciousness to self-awareness. The *opus* of transformation begins in the *prima materia* – the chaotic, undifferentiated mass and mess, often colored black, that is in need of transformation. The first stage that is differentiated out from the the *prima materia*—the *nigredo*—is also black. If the *prima materia* is uncreated and unformed, the chaotic potential of the unconscious, the *nigredo* is characterized by depression, desolation, grief, mourning, disintegration and psychic death; it is often represented in alchemical treatises by black crows, skeletons, and skulls. In practice these two beginning stages are often inter-twined. Following the *nigredo* comes the *albedo*, an internal state of realiza-tion of new attitudes risen from the ashes of the *nigredo*. It is an internal state of rebirth, of purity and innocence—whiteness without the oppositional nature Hillman says is essential to the color. But although the *albedo* is a great achievement, it requires to be "reddened"—given life and blood. In the final stage of the *rubedo*, the realizations gained from suffering and reflection come to have effects in the outer world. Thus this three-stage model of transformation allows us to escape the trap of static, oppositional thinking and makes room for movement and change.

Black as mirror

On a wall in a quiet corner of the Museo Nacional de Antropología in México City hangs a *tezcatl*, a polished obsidian disk about seven inches in diameter. This is the Smoking Mirror of the Black Tezcatlipoca, White Tezcatlipoca Quetzalcóatl's twin brother. Along with their siblings Blue Tezcatlipoca Huitzilopochtli and Red Tezcatlipoca Xipe Totec, they are the children of the androgynous, self-birthed deity Ometecuhtli/Omecihuatl. In Toltec mythology, the four are related to the four directions and are responsible for the creation of all the other gods, the world, and humankind. As the 'Lord of Fatality', Black Tezcatlipoca is the god of providence, rul-ership, the North, the earth, divination, sorcery, temptation, conflict, deceit, judgment, war, hurricanes, beauty, the night and its creatures, especially the jaguar, who has the capacity to pass between the earth and the underworld. A hymn describes Black Tezcatlipoca as a poet and a scribe as well as the world's creator and destroyer. A trickster, he lost his foot by using it as bait to catch the crocodilian earth monster Cipactli, whose body became the land. Black Tezcatlipoca and Quetzalcóatl fought one another as they created and destroyed four successive worlds, until at last they co-created the fifth world, which is ours.

Walking up to the mirror, you see yourself as a dimly perceived presence in its intensely black space. The Mexica (Aztec) believed that black obsidian had spiritual significance. In the obsidian mirror's reflection, Black Tezcatlipoca looked back at the person looking into it, and the black reflection could heal blackness of heart and soul. Thus the obsidian mirror was an alchemical medicine in which the poison—the blackness—was also the panacea, the healing substance. The Mexica used obsidian as a medicine to ward off evil spirits, capture souls, and divine the future. John Dee, alchemist and Elizabeth I of England's court astrologer, owned such a mirror.

In contrast to Black Tezcatlipoca, White Tezcatlpoca, or Quetzalcóatl (Feathered Serpent), is the god of the dawn, the West, the sun and the wind, beauty and light, learning and craftsmanship, wisdom, justice, and mercy. He invented books and the calendar. Associated with rulers and priests, Quetzalcóatl gives maize to the people. Mexican author Juan Villoro tells this story about Quetzalcóatl and the Smoking Mirror:

> An enlightened god, Quetzalcoatl lived for knowledge, but he did not know his own face. That shortcoming gave rise to a curious divine dispute. The pre-Hispanic sky was a stage for gods in conflict. Tezcatlipoca, the Lord of Fatality, had a smoking obsidian mirror—whoever looked into it would gaze upon their inevitable destiny. In order to defeat Quetzalcoatl, Tezcatlipoca made him look at his own face. On the polished obsidian surface, that harmony-seeking god beheld an aberration: a confusing creature, part bird and part reptile. Horrified by his image, he threw down the mirror and fled from the people who had venerated him. The mirror remained buried like a time capsule, waiting to acquire another meaning.
>
> (Villoro 2021, n.p.)

The mirror of archetypal black inflicted a necessary loss, shattering Quetzalcóatl's clean, white self-image. Unable to handle this defeat, the god turned away from self-knowledge. Part aerial spirit, part chthonic deity, whiteness runs away because it cannot understand its own completeness-in-difference.

The self, says Octavio Paz, is 'a lost being that can only recognize himself [sic] in "all the others that we are"'. According to Villoro, Paz and others have used this legend to express the need for Mexicans to accept their contradictory natures—to overcome the complex of being different and to 'establish a dialogue of plurality with other cultures, [of] equity among differences'. Villoro ends his essay with the words: '[o]ur perception of ourselves depends on what is "other", to the same extent that the future is nourished by another era' (Villoro 2021, n.p.). To escape from black-and-white, "us vs. them" thinking, we must see ourselves in our completeness. Without knowing the complexity of our own nature—part soaring spirit, part chthonic creature, part light and part shadow, part white, part black—we cannot experience 'equity among differences'. Quetzalcóatl must see that he is as much serpent as bird. The myth asserts that there can be no 'dialogue of plurality' without this self-recognition which also allows us to recognize, in each other person we encounter, a completeness composed of differences.

The black mirror, mirroring back our blackness, offers an image by means of which the too-white side of the racial complex is asked to undergo the process of the *nigredo*. Hillman describes how the *nigredo*'s 'depression, fixations, obsessions, and a general blackening of mood and vision' may initiate necessary change by dissolving no-longer-viable structures of consciousness. Its blackening negates 'the light of knowledge, the attachment to solar consciousness as far-seeing prediction, or the feeling that phenomena can be understood. Black dissolves meaning and the hope for meaning.' Blackness breaks down fixed states by falling apart, by decomposition, by grinding down (Hillman 1997/2010, loc. 1693–97). 'Like cures like; we cure the *nigredo* by becoming, as the texts say, blacker than black—archetypally black, and thereby no longer colored by all-too-human prejudices of color' (Hillman 1997/2010, loc. 1842–44).

The Smoking Mirror has long awaited another time to do its work. Recognizing this duality in ourselves requires that we—both individually and collectively—gaze into our psyche's mirror in order to unhook, from the others we have required to carry them, our projections of the archetypal qualities of black. Then our encounters with others can be based on 'equity among differences', no matter the outer colors.

Remembering

Do not trust the eraser. Prefer
crossed out, scribbled over monuments
to something once thought correct.
Instead: colors, transparencies
track changes, versions, iterations.
How else might you return
after discards, attempts
and mis takes, to your
original genius?

(King 2022)

King's poem reminds us that we cannot and should not try to erase the story of racism. The poem also provides possible ways forward. King suggests that, without erasing historical records of abuse and trauma, we may be able to cross out incorrect assumptions as we write a new story. We may be able to use 'colors, transparencies'—perhaps the both/and ambi-valences of red—to return to an 'original genius' that allows for the future of equity and plurality Villoro hopes for.

Jung tells us that we do not get rid of complexes, at best becoming more conscious of them, through the blackening offered by the Smoking Mirror. We cannot erase our culture's history of mistreating Blacks. Instead, the outer restitution and inner healing of racial self-hatred require working sensitively in recognition of racial cultural complexes that reside within both white and black persons. The image reflected in the Smoking Mirror depends upon the person looking into it and his or her position(s) in the cultural complex. For white persons, as for Quetzalcóatl, the mirror may show us 'all the others that we are'—the amalgam of light and shadow we have wanted to keep separate. The black surface may reflect our internal blackness, grounding us in our own interior differences and helping us to work toward equity among them.

For analysts, seeing the double face of our sometimes too-good self-valuation may help to bring our own 'completeness-in-difference' into the work. Like

Quetzalcóatl, we need to see both the high-minded, well-intentioned and the dark sides of ourselves. The mirror also demands that we remember the ways our experiences 'embody, or reflect, or are relevant to aspects of the "patient's" experience, … [and that w]henever there is an experience of countertransference, there is uncertainty about whose "stuff" it is' (Samuels 1993, loc. 929, 944). Our connection to our own history is as important as the patient's.

The need for Black patients to address the intergenerational trauma of fear, invisibility, and self-hatred that many carry in their bodies and psyches takes particular forms. Black analysts have written eloquently about the healing needed amidst the traumas of racism in the aftermath of slavery. Mirroring of this historical trauma as well as of the very personhood of Black people is especially needed. Samuel Kimbles (2014) describes the 'invisibility complex' that is a core part of Black identity in America:

> [T]he unconsciously supremacist "white" could, by simply averting his or her gaze, arrogating the right to direct it as he or she chose, destroy the "person of color" as someone who didn't deserve being looked at as one would a fully human subject. What remained was stereotyping, prejudices, devaluing, and so on, as the only forms of mirroring that some whites would afford blacks and that blacks would receive. As we all now know, thanks in part to [Ralph] Ellison's brilliance [in *Invisible Man*], that starvation diet of mirroring leads to the creation of a self (system) that divides the races beyond any possibility of mutuality … . It reflects a breakdown in the relationship between humans as subjects (accepting one's own reality) and the reality of the other (as equal and legitimate).
>
> (Kimbles 2014, p. 27)

Kimbles describes how analytic work can address this sense of invisibility by holding up a different mirror from the one American culture has provided Black persons. By such witnessing, we can not only make room for the patient to reflect on his or her history, but also 'become part of the process of making history through our relationship to the patient. Indeed, we become part of their history' (ibid., p. 26). But Andrew Samuels cautions that, in making space for recalling history, '[t]he therapist is not an authority or teacher who has a priori knowledge of the psychological implications of the client's ethnic and cultural background'. Our concern should not be with defining difference, but with 'the experience of difference'. 'Each patient may be seen as struggling toward a recognition, expression and celebration of his or her own difference' (Samuels 1993, pp. 54, 158).

Fanny Brewster writes movingly about the fear, shame, invisibility, self-suppression, and self-vanishing contained in the racial complexes of Black persons:

When a racial complex is triggered by a sense of worthlessness that appears in behaviors or feelings of shame and being undeserving of good, can we not help but see patterns of self-destruction. Who speaks for our worth and how do we better learn the inner language of self-value? … [C]lients of color will be engaged in clinical work oftentimes with expressed or unexpressed/unidentified ideas that have to do with their racial complexes. Most times, it is essential to work with these patients in helping them identify their cultural racial complexes so that they can learn how to release themselves from feelings of guilt, depression and anger.

(Brewster 2019, loc. 788, 2,139)

The invisibility complex described by Kimbles may be constellated in analysis, especially when a therapist appears uncomfortable discussing racial trauma. Yet along with Samuels, Brewster emphasizes the need to work at the patient's pace:

It is important that the individual, if possible, is allowed to work at their own pace of integration. Therefore, the decision to talk about racial issues should be guided by the readiness of the individual and the group, but sometimes that decision is taken away by unconscious processes such as transference and countertransference evoked in the here and now. The aim needs to be about understanding why what is happening at that particular moment.

(Brewster 2019, loc. 2,108)

In 'Wheel of Fire' (2013), Brewster decries the negative description of Black culture and ideas, and the 'perpetuation of insidious racism within our American collective', emphasizing its destructive effects on the psychological well-being of both black and white persons (Brewster 2013, p. 76). She makes a plea for a more nuanced and positive image of African American culture:

A positive cultural consciousness means having an awareness of the attributes of one's own cultural heritage and that of others without being predisposed to negative assumptions and projections about what forms this heritage, whether we are speaking of linguistics (Ebonics), food (soul)—or of music, spiritual beliefs, and other ethnic dynamics. Positive African American consciousness includes a respectful regard for all aspects of the sociological and historical African American life experience without consistent and predominantly negative bias.

(Brewster 2013, p. 77)

Here the Smoking Mirror can call us forward toward a place where the archetypal might provide relief from the cultural. Withdrawing the "flat black" of projection does not by itself afford the material for a whole self-image. But the unconscious helps through corrective images of blackness in dreams. Drawing on the power and intensity of archetypal imagery of the color black—going beyond depression, despair, shadow figure, devil, or fearful darkness to the potentiality and mystery of being and becoming—is a way of thinking about being black that loosens up the cultural complex, freeing us from the clamped jaws of present-tense experience to a larger sense of self.

To those who can sustain its reflection, the mirror of the unconscious, like the Black Tezcatlipoca's obsidian mirror, reveals this wider, deeper, more complexly-whole self. As Baldwin says:

> [T]he question of color, especially in this country, operates to hide the graver questions of the self. That is precisely why what we like to call "the Negro problem" is so tenacious in American life, and so dangerous. But my own experience proves to me that the connection between American whites and blacks is far deeper and more passionate than any of us like to think. ... The questions which one asks oneself begin, at last, to illuminate the world, and become one's key to the experience of others. One can only face in others what one can face in oneself.
>
> (Baldwin 1961/1993, p. xii)

The mirror is a cure for invisibility and a source for envisioning completeness-in-difference. It offers a reflection that fosters healing of the ego's relationship to the Self's inner guiding principle.

Notes

1 The shooter stated on social media that 'all black people are replacers just by existing in White countries' (Kendi 2022).
2 'The baby, assailed by eyes, ears, nose, skin, and entrails at once, feels it all as one great blooming, buzzing confusion' (James 1890, p. 488).
3 At the extreme, as described by the historian Joel Kovel, white Americans have feared to be "polluted" by touching Black persons (1970; in Adams 1996, pp. 132–33).
4 The latest evidence of the evolution of skin color differences reverses this etiology. The human groups who migrated to northern Europe from Africa with dark skin lost their dark color in response to northern climatic conditions, because lighter skin absorbs UV wavelengths, necessary for the synthesis of Vitamin D from the oils of the skin, more readily (Gibbons 2015). This theory posits dark skin as the normative condition, from which light skin is a deviation.

References

Adams, M. J. (1996). *The Multicultural Imagination: "Race", Color, and the Unconscious*. London and New York: Routledge.
Baldwin, J. A. (1961/1993). *Nobody Knows My Name: More Notes of a Native Son*. New York: Vintage.

Baldwin, J. A. (1962/1998). 'Down at the cross'. *The Fire Next Time*. Republished in James Baldwin: Collected Essays, selected by Toni Morrison. New York: The Library of America.

Baldwin, J. A. & Luster, O. (1964). 'Take this hammer'. Richard O. Moore, producer and director. National Educational Television, February 4.

Boyle, R. (1664). *Experiments and Considerations Touching Colours*. London: Henry Herringman.

Brewster, F. (2013). 'Wheel of fire: the African American dreamer and cultural consciousness'. *Jung Journal: Culture & Psyche*, 7, 1, 70–87.

Brewster, F. (2019). *The Racial Complex: A Jungian Perspective on Culture and Race*. Oxford UK: Routledge.

Circlot, J. E. (1962/1971). *A Dictionary of Symbols*, trans. Jack Sage. 2nd ed. London: Routledge and Kegan Paul, Ltd.

Cooper, J. C. (1978). *An Illustrated Encyclopaedia of Traditional Symbols*. London: Thames & Hudson.

Dehai, H., Jing, X. & Dinghau, Z. (2018). *Illustrated Myths & Legends of China: The Ages of Chaos and Heroes*, trans. T. Blishen. New York: Better Link Press.

Douglas, M. (1966/2002). *Purity and Danger*. Oxford, UK: Routledge and Kegan Paul.

Dumézil, G. (1945). *Rituels Indo-européens à Rome*. Paris: C. Klincksieck.

von Franz, M-L. (1972/1995). *Creation Myths*. Rev. ed. Boulder, CO: Shambhala Publications, Inc.

Gass, W. H. (1976/2014). *On Being Blue: A Philosophical Inquiry*. New York: New York Review Books.

Gibbons, A. (2015). 'How Europeans evolved white skin'. *Science*, April 2. Retrieved from https://www.science.org/content/article/how-europeans-evolved-white-skin (accessed 2022-06-15).

Goldin, O. (2015). 'The Pythagorean table of opposites, symbolic classification, and Aristotle'. *Science in Context*, 28, 2, 171–193.

Hillman, J. (1986). 'Notes on white supremacy: essaying an archetypal account of historical events'. *Spring*.

Hillman, J. (1997/2010). 'The seduction of black'. Uniform Edition of the Writings of James Hillman. Vol. 5, Alchemical Psychology. Putnam, CT: Spring Publications, Inc. *Originally published in* Haiti: Or The Psychology of Black, Spring 61, October, ed. J. Hillman, C. Boer & J. Bertoia.

Houck-Loomis, T. (2022). Personal communication, 27 September.

James, W. (1890). *The Principles of Psychology*. New York: Henry Holt and Company.

Jobes, G. (1962). *Dictionary of Mythology, Folklore and Symbols*. 3 vols. Lanham, MD: The Scarecrow Press, Inc.

Jordan, W. D. (1968). *White over Black: American Attitudes toward the Negro, 1550–1812*. New York: W. W. Norton and Company.

Jung, C. G. (1960). 'A review of the complex theory'. The Structure and Dynamics of the Psyche. CW 8. 2nd ed. Princeton, NJ: Princeton University Press.

Kendi, I. X. (2016). *Stamped from the Beginning: The Definitive History of Racist Ideas in America*. New York: Bold Type Books.

Kendi, I. X. (2022). 'The double terror of being black in America'. *The Atlantic*, May 20.

Kimbles, S. (2014). *Phantom Narratives: The Unseen Contributions of Culture to Psyche*. Lanham, MD: Rowman & Littlefield.

King, R. S. (2022). 'Do not trust the eraser'. *Poem-a-Day*, July 1. The Academy of American Poets. Retrieved from https://poets.org/poem/do-not-trust-eraser?mc_cid=6f68705dd2&mc_eid=7e33c52111 (accessed 2022-07-04).

Kovel, J. (1970). *White Racism: A Psychohistory*. New York: Pantheon.

Locke, J. (1690/2019). *An Essay Concerning Human Understanding in Four Books*. Whithorn, Newton Steward, Scotland: Anodos Books.

McDaniel, S. (2020). 'Were the ancient Greeks and Romans white?' Retrieved from https://talesoftimesforgotten.com/2020/09/30/were-the-ancient-greeks-and-romans-white/ (accessed 2022-07-31).

McNatt, G. (2007). 'Unmasking the meaning behind color in African art'. *Baltimore Sun*, April 17. Retrieved from https://www.baltimoresun.com/news/bs-xpm-2007-04-18-0704180243-story.html (accessed 2022-07-11).

Menakem, R. (2017). *My Grandmother's Hands: Racialized Trauma and the Pathway to Mending Our Hearts and Bodies*. Las Vegas: Central Recovery Press.

Monier-Williams, M. (1899/2005). *A Sanskrit–English Dictionary: Etymologically and Philologically Arranged with Special Reference to Cognate Indo-European Languages. Reprinted*. Delhi: Motilal Banarsidass.

Montagu, A. (1945). *Man's Most Dangerous Myth: The Fallacy of Race*. New York: Columbia University Press.

Newton, I. (1672). 'Mr Isaac Newton's answer to some considerations [of Robert Hooke] upon his doctrine of light and colors'. *Philosophical Transactions of the Royal Society*, 88, 18 November, 5084–5103. Retrieved from https://www.newtonproject.ox.ac.uk/view/texts/normalized/NATP00028 (accessed 2022-07-19).

Palmiotto, P. (2016). 'Jung's theory of complexes and the neurosciences'. Retrieved from https://www.immaginipsiche.it/2016/12/19/jungs-theories-of-complexes-and-the-neurosciences/ (accessed 2022-06-27).

Pastoureau, M. (2009). *Black: The History of a Color*, trans. J. Gladding. Princeton, NJ: Princeton University Press.

Russell-Cole, K., Wilson, M. & Hall, R. E. (2013). *The Color Complex: The Politics of Skin Color in a New Millennium*. Rev. ed. New York: Anchor Books.

Samuels, A. (1993). *The Political Psyche*. Oxford, UK: Routledge.

Singer, T. & Kimbles, S. L. (2004). 'Introduction'. *The Cultural Complex*, ed. T. Singer & S. L. Kimbles. New York: Brunner-Routledge.

Smedley, A. & Smedley, B. (2012). *Race in North America: Origin and Evolution of a Worldview*. Boulder, CO: Westview Press.

Turner, V. (1967). 'Color classification in Ndembu ritual'. *The Forest of Symbols: Aspects of Ndembu Ritual*. Ithaca, NY: Cornell University Press.

Villoro, J. (2021). 'The obsidian mirror: Mexican archaeology and literature in dialogue'. *Harvard Divinity Bulletin*, Autumn/Winter. Retrieved from: https://bulletin.hds.harvard.edu/the-obsidian-mirror/ (accessed 2022-07-11).

de Vries, A. & de Vries, A. (1974/2004). *Elsevier's Dictionary of Symbols and Imagery*. 2nd enlarged ed. Bingley, UK: Emerald Group Publishing Limited.

Warbuton, D. (2014). 'Ancient color categories'. *Encyclopedia of Color Science and Technology*. New York: Springer Science + Business Media.

Wilkerson, I. (2020). *Caste: The Origins of Our Discontents*. New York: Random House.

Chapter 4

On Failings

Sherry Salman

Introduction

Among the Baule people of the Republic of Côte d'Ivoire, Africa, human experience remains linked to the ancestral spirit world, or *blolo*, the 'Village of Truth' (LaGamma 2000). Always influencing the fate of the living, the Village of Truth comprises of the present extended generation of villagers, the next generation not born yet, and five generations of ancestors. The oldest of these ancestors merges with the forces of nature and the gods, becoming oracular spirits.

From a psychological perspective, the discipline and culture of analytical psychology exists on the cusp of a Village of Truth, with one foot still in and one foot moving out. Jung is now our ancestral spirit, a spirit whom we consult on a regular basis to understand deep psychological processes. We look to Jung to discover the creation myths of our origination, and, more importantly, we look to Jung to assist us as we discover new beginnings for next generations—new beginnings that speak to both the spirit of the times and the spirit of the depths. Jung's work still offers a portal into the archetypal elements of psychological process, a way into the ancestral mythopoetic mind, the bedrock container that holds us as we relate our theories and practice to the spirit of the times.

At the same time, it is always disorienting, even frightening, to leave the Village of Truth and discover that as one's ancestral spirit merges with nature and the mythic mind, its outlines are no longer easy to discern. As we gain distance and perspective some of those lines no longer plumb true. Jung has become protean, a shapeshifter impossible to pin down, and no amount of heroic effort—whether that be hanging on to tradition or smashing idols—is going to pin that spirit down. Nor should it.

This chapter begins by discussing ways in which Jung failed to apply several of his analytic ideas to himself as he encountered what was other in himself, and, actual other people and their traditions in Africa. These failures were intertwined with a kind of twin birth: the first was Jung's projection of anima-loaded 'primitivity' onto others while at the same time romanticizing

DOI: 10.4324/9781003311447-5

the psychology of 'archaic man' (Jung 1931/1964). The second birth was the myth of consciousness, a story that elevated human consciousness to the position of co-creator of the world (Jung 1963/1989). In Africa Jung was hyper stimulated by his experiences, and, began to discover his own life's mythic map, a multi-dimensional map that found its most sophisticated and creative differentiation in the alchemical model of psychological development. Jung went to Africa in 1925, and it was truly the trip of a lifetime, an outer journey running parallel to the intense inner experiences chronicled in *The Red Book* that spanned the years 1913–1930.

It was also a trip that generated failures. It is odious and arduous work to acknowledge Jung's prejudicial projections onto Africans, projections that he never quite recollected. Some of these resulted, for example, in the biased and abortive reaction of interpreting a black-skinned figure in the dream of a white person as a shadow figure—or the opposite, as the apotheosis of natural wisdom. We also cringe in the face of the Eurocentric myth of consciousness that struck Jung on the Athai Plains, a myth that transmogrified into the 'white man's burden' of bringing consciousness to the benighted. It is a sad state of affairs that still cries out for mourning and action on all fronts. Jung actually loathed imperialism, and his recognition of a dynamic relationship to the mythopoetic psyche as *sine qua non* of individuated life has endured. However, the spirit of our times calls out for recollecting these racialized projections. History is never really forgotten, it exists in us until we come to terms with it, with the ancestors, the ghosts, the dead, and the events of the past that are alive right now and having effects everywhere. The spirit of our times aims to give voice to what has been speechless or deemed inferior, to witness and mourn what seems unbearable, to give space and silence for narratives and symbols of identity to form and re-form, to undergo the great tragic drama of mortification. We can choose to live as greening cemeteries, the dead and wounded within us alive and fertile, providing inexhaustible compost for growth. Or, we become the housing for what psychoanalysts Abraham and Torok (1994) have called 'psychic crypts' wherein traumatic wounds and history are not merely buried or repressed but *are never actually experienced at all.*

On a personal note, I had read some of Jung's work before beginning my training in 1979. His writings on the psychic constitution of black skinned people, the overdetermination of the anima idea and the consequent bizarre statements about women all made my hair stand on end. With the hubris of the young, it all struck me as so disgusting that I almost derailed the surrender to my vocation. But I put my misgivings to the side and moved forward, although they haunted me in ways that I could not quite explain, other than acknowledging that some of Jung's sentiments were, in fact, a grievous failure. What I failed to grasp in my youth was that the failure to recognize or fully understand moments of crucial importance such as those that affected Jung deeply in Africa, are not only personally or culturally determined. Some failures are also archetypal and capable of inducing a mortification and mourning that flower into the reconstitution of a larger personality. I did not fully understand that the cycle of failure, mortification, and, reintegration is itself a mythic motif.[1] If fully suffered, that failure can generate a deeply reflective consciousness.

Was Jung himself mortified by some of what he wrote about the primitive mind and African people, or by the perhaps defensive inflation coloring his elevation of conscious man as the co-creator of the world that Africa inspired in him? It would seem mostly not. The chapter on 'Travels' in Jung's auto-biography *Memories, Dreams, Reflections* (*MDR*), a chapter largely about his African safari, was left to stand as is for publication, with all its distortions and mistakes intact. They were not reflected upon, even though Jung's safari took place some thirty-five years before his death.

In the poem "Last Night as I Was Sleeping", Antonio Machado wrote, 'I dreamt last night oh marvelous error, that there were honeybees here inside my heart, making sweet honey from my old failures' (Machado 1983). It is left to present and future generations of analysts to undergo the proper mortificatio and make honey from the errors and failures of our ancestor. It is work to be undertaken with an open heart and a loving mind, and, with an acceptance of failings as an indispensable ingredient of individuation and cultural progress. To restore our particular psychological culture, we have to open the crypts and put ourselves in order without losing the symbolic sensibility that understands certain failures to be mythic as well as cultural illnesses.

This chapter ends with a discussion of how we engage with failings from a depth symbolic perspective, including the failings that our patients bring into analysis, and with the subversive tricksters-inspired failures of analysis itself. For 'Failures', as the ancestor wrote in 'The Psychology of the Transference', 'are priceless experiences because they not only open the way to a better truth but force us to modify our views and methods' (Jung 1946/1985, para 73). They also place the crucial challenge for individuals and communities right on the table: how we act in relation to our own dirt.

In and out of the bath in Africa

Before his safari to Africa in 1925, a very nervous Jung was consulting the *I Ching* daily. One of his traveling companions had suddenly withdrawn from the trip, the wife of another fell seriously ill with depression, the funding was threatened with collapse (Burleson 2005, pp. 15–26). Quite worried, as the departure date drew closer, Jung cast hexagram #53, 'Development' (Gradual Progress) with the following moving line,

> The wild goose gradually draws near the plateau. The man goes forth and does not return. The woman carries a child but does not bring it forth. Misfortune. It furthers one to fight off robbers.

> (Wilhelm 1950/1967, p. 206)

Jung went to Africa despite darkening clouds, interpreting the oracle as both a good omen signaling progress, and a warning of danger. The danger, as it appeared to Jung, was of not returning, of dying, or of going mad, of going too far, of transgressing too many internal boundaries, and, as stated elsewhere, of 'going black' (Jung 1930/1964, para 967). He was certain that he needed to protect his European personality. However, like a good oracle, the *I Ching* presaged his failure to withdraw his shadow and anima projections onto Africans and Africa, and the retreat into his persona—the woman carries a child but does not bring it forth. Misfortune.

Jung's interpretation of what was dangerous in 1925 was very peculiar, considering that one of the opening salvos in *The Red Book* had been a vision experienced in 1913 of the murder of Siegfried, an Aryan hero who appears in old Norse and Germanic myths (Jung 2009, p. 241). This vision seemed to announce the self-inflicted death of a collective ego ideal in Jung's psyche. Moreover, later in the *Red Book*, Jung's soul speaks to him about madness

> Have you recognized your madness and do you admit it? Have you noticed that all your foundations are completely mired in madness? Do you not want to recognize your madness and welcome it in a friendly manner? You wanted to accept everything. So accept madness too. Let the light of your madness shine, and it will suddenly dawn on you. Madness is not to be despised and not to be feared, but instead you should give it life ... you should not spurn madness since it makes up such a great part of your nature ... . Madness is itself a special form of the spirit, since life itself is full of craziness and at bottom utterly illogical.
>
> (Jung 2009, p. 298)

Jung went to Africa for at least two expressed reasons: to find a vantage point outside of himself from which to critique the alienated Western psyche, and to pose to himself, 'the rather embarrassing question: What is going to happen to Jung the psychologist in the wilds of Africa?' (Jung 1963/1989, p. 273). It seemed that Jung both valorized what he felt in Africa and feared being seduced and disoriented by the enchantment and madness that he explicitly courted in Africa. He allowed some of the madness in, and he also shut it out via un-recollected projections and othering. This is evident in his somewhat confessionary, sad, and maddening statement, 'I have not been led by any kind of wisdom; I have been led by dreams, like any primitive. I am ashamed to say so, but I am as primitive as any nigger because I do not know' (Jung 1939/1989, para 674).

As the power and the projections of the unconscious onto Africans became increasingly charged, another vision took hold of Jung, one that was directly compensatory to the story about the wisdom of the primitive unconscious. Not a pluralistic vision of the multiplicity of unconscious process, the second story was a monomyth about the primacy of consciousness,[2] a myth about human consciousness completing the creation of the world. In *MDR*, Jung wrote about a formative experience in Africa that occurred during the same period; that he was most impressed by the archaic world that he imagined he resided there, pristine, undisturbed, and also, inferior. As he surveyed the Athai Plains of Kenya, Jung thought

> Now I knew what it was, and knew even more: that man is indispensable for the completion of creation; that, in fact, he himself is the second creator of the world, who alone has given to the world its objective existence— without which, unheard, unseen, silently eating, giving birth, dying, heads nodding through hundreds of millions of years, it would have gone on in the profoundest night of non-being down to its unknown end. Human consciousness created objective existence and meaning, and man found his indispensable place in the great process of being.
>
> (Jung 1963/1989, p. 256)

On the one hand this astonishing statement foreshadows Jung's adoption of alchemy as a roadmap for individuation, i.e., what Nature leaves imperfect, the Art perfects. However, many today would be painfully chagrined by this privileging of human consciousness and the many shadows that follow in its wake: a perverse interiority and consequent othering, a destructive narcissism and cultural imperialism that too often expressed itself as the white man's burden, and the failure to contextualize an archetypal experience within the cultural framework in which it was expressed. In line with this last point regarding contextualization, and even more unsettling, Europeans, it seemed, being at the pinnacle of psychological development carry within their psyches the whole history of humankind from the primitive (instinctual, animal-like, dark, lower) to the civilized (differentiated, European-like, light, higher). Like a mistaken phylogenetic time-traveler, convinced that ontogeny recapitulates phylogeny,[3] Jung wrote:

> In the collective unconscious, you are the same as a man of another race. You have the same archetypes, just as you have, like him, eyes, a heart, and so on. It does not matter that his skin is black. It matters to a certain extent, sure enough—he probably has a whole layer less than you. The different strata of the mind correspond to the history of the races.
>
> (Jung 1935/1976, para 93)

All of this is misguided and particularly racist if it advocates that Europeans, and perhaps their 'affable but slightly imbecilic' cousins, the Americans,[4] could understand Africans better than Africans could understand themselves.

While elevating the myth of consciousness that he seemed to discover on the Athai Plains, Jung also romanticized, valued—and sometimes disparaged—the 'primitive' psyche: the world of fairies, archaic man, mana, the bush soul, all the magical fields of awareness dominated by *participation mystique* that would later give rise to a more mature and unprejudiced synchronistic sensibility. The oscillation and tension between these two states of mind was baked into Jung, perhaps echoed in his awareness of his own personalities One and Two. These two fields of awareness and their parallel development were portals for developing the methods of archetypal amplification and active imagination: the first a conscious elaboration and systematized collection of archetypal themes across history and cultures, the second, the living experience of the mythopoetic psyche. Nowhere was the tension between them more pronounced and unresolved than what is evident in Jung's confused—and as it turned out, quite mad—conclusions about Africans in Africa.

Regressive restoration of the persona

A regressive restoration of the persona fell upon Jung in Africa, a halt in growth, a failure of integration, and a state often characterized by rigid othering of projected contents. This was likely due to fear of ego collapse, of being swallowed in identification with the collective psyche, becoming lost in the belly of the whale, in this case, in what he felt to be the darkness of Africa. Writing on regressive restoration, Jung informs us:

> The regressive restoration of the persona is a possible course only for the man who owes the critical failure of his life to his own inflatedness. With diminished personality, he turns back to the measure he can fill.
>
> (Jung 1953/1972, para 259)

There is a poignancy to this, as Jung deeply wanted to embark on the hero's journey and the renewal that comes with surrender to the unknown aspects of his psychology. Perhaps the glamour of that desire was the inflation, but it was not to be. Of all the critiques of Jung, the one of racism is perhaps the most critical, the one most in need of understanding and dismantling, as the spirit of our times demands.

Jung the psychologist got lost in Africa. As he got closer to re-visioning the creative significance of the mythopoetic mind, he also began to interpret his own dreams defensively. The infamous barber dream, the only dream Jung had in Africa featuring a black-skinned person, was taken as a warning and cemented his conviction that he was too close to the brink. In the dream, a Black man who Jung associated to his American barber in Tennessee,

> ... was holding a tremendous, red-hot curling iron to my head, intending to make my hair kinky—that is, to give me Negro hair. I could already feel the painful heat, and awoke with a sense of terror.
>
> (Jung 1963/1989, p. 272)

Afraid of 'going black under the skin' (ibid., p. 245), which Jung considered to be a spiritual peril for all uprooted Europeans, Jung decided that an 'interior line was being successfully secured within my dreams' (ibid., p. 273). Gone was the symbolic perspective that would have recognized an initiation ritual, a trial by fire. Instead, this is exactly when Jung decided that 'my European personality must under all circumstances be preserved intact' (ibid.).

Making matters worse, Jung heard only one dream from an African during the five months he was there—a bad sign if ever there was one. Jung explained this barrenness of dreams told to him by Africans as due to a fear within the African of their soul being stolen, and to the ubiquitous 'English problem'[5] (ibid., p. 265). Despite the *I Ching* reading he failed to understand what was happening as resonating with archetypal or even subjective factors in himself, except to wonder whether his desire to journey to Africa had been a desire to escape from the tense and charged atmosphere at home.

Failings in analysis and trickster dynamics

Failures in analytic journeys have usually been attributed to a host of ills: bad technique, wrong diagnoses, countertransference, advanced or youthful age of the patient, negative therapeutic reaction, intractable idealization, narcissistic or borderline personality disorder, weak ego, intense early trauma, empathic failures, and lack of attunement, and what may be called the general nonfulfillment of expectations on either side—often defined as the patient not being or feeling cured. There are failures to go deep, and failures to know when not to. Failures to keep silent, and failures to feel and to think and to act. There are failures to adhere to one's theory and correct practice or even one's belief about analytic success or failure. The list is inexhaustible and the punishment for failure often severe: orthodox retrenchment in theory and ideas about unanalyzable patients, a negative inflation, guiltiness or shame, a defeated retreat into fate or a grandiose contempt for it, and a debilitating lack of faith in the whole analytic enterprise that sometimes precipitates a sado-masochistic acting out against one's patients, oneself, or, against other failed analysts. As analyst Judith Vida wrote in *The Indispensable "Difficult Event"*, 'When failure is a capital crime in the unconscious, execution awaits' (Reppen & Schulman 2018, p. 18).

Surely, we do not aspire to sentence patients or analysts for the failings and transgressions that come into analysis. Those failures, both past and present, often contain *prima materia* for the work when understood prospectively. We try to not get stuck in condemning parents, life events, trauma, and, other 'just so' occasions and circumstances of living. We understand analysis to be a tricky and subversive enterprise, full or wrong turns, detours, backwards and forwards movement, and especially surprises. There are times of intense generativity and times of rest, times when the persona is restored regressively and times when it is renewed and expanded. Just when things seem clear and consolidated, suddenly they are not, and rogue or newly born elements make their presence known.

As mythology and history suggest, failure comes right along with subversive moves, if only to the extent that one has failed to adhere to the psychological or societal status quo by being ill. Or better yet, failure is the first sign that collective and cultural ideals are being actively deconstructed. Perhaps best of all, failures and transgressions into new psychological territory can be the great transformers of culture. As cultural critic Lewis Hyde wrote, 'Trickster makes this world' (1998).

At one time the *Oxford English Dictionary* defined "to fail" as simply "to die" (Winchester 1998). When viewed prospectively death points to renewal after a period of incubation and rot. What is on the table now for Jungian communities is how we will act in relation to our own dirt and rot. That dirt may be outright or misbegotten prejudices. That dirt may be the failure to teach Jung's work as a living symbolic process instead of dogma. That dirt may be a failure to remain in alignment with what the spirit of the times has brought into focus. Jung is now an ancestor, a spirit, even a culture that tends toward drinking from the inexhaustible spring of imagination and mythopoetic thinking—a culture whose methods help differentiate between 'the fantasies spun into repetition by complexes and the "true imagination" of psyche's archetypal trajectories' (Salman 2006). But Jung the man is dead, and, his dirt is coming fully into view. If left unexplored in the full light of community the dirt can poison the well. It is not that hard to become a footnote in history.

Culturally, it is not a coincidence that the sharp focus on the rot of racism at the core of so much of American culture is occurring alongside the tearing down and failures of institutions of all sorts. When one isn't looking at the rigidity of prevailing structures or paying attention to what is standing at the margins in plain sight, hungry and pressing for inclusion, we can be sure that trickster dynamics will erupt from the unconscious. This is a "just so" archetypal dynamic. For example, a case could be made that the failure to pay attention to what was hungry on "the other side" provoked the intense eruption of the hallucinogenic inspired sea change of the 1960s that ran riotously over nuclear family values, the segregation of women and black skinned people, and the esteemed stability of the 1950s. Or, viewed from the other "other side", the rioting and shooting in venerated government buildings, and of children and ethnic minorities in the 21st century suggests a failure to have paid attention to what and whom had been hungry and left out of the financial and techno-inspired spiritless culture of the preceding years. Trickster dynamics have a very good nose for failures and the dynamic does not choose sides. It is a wired-in mechanism that corrects for failures of imagination and complacent rigidity wherever those exist. Older cultures gave time for the throwdowns and reversals that failures inspire and that trickster dynamics provide by building them into their cultural calendars and ceremonies. In the USA, we have a paltry and ineffective April Fool's Day. The only way to slip through the cracks in the rubble that accumulates as trickster takes apart persona ideals *is to find ways to ritualize our own disruption and renewal.*

A conclusion

Jung was fooled in Africa, likely by the people living there, and by his own psyche. He longed for the disruption that Africa and Africans would induce in him, but in many ways, he failed to fully transgress. His failure to apply his own ideas about persona, shadow, and anima possession to himself turned out to be a moment of crucial importance. It would take him years to work himself at least partly out of those failures. Whether these were failures of nerve, a deeply held fear of the ethnic other, a seizure by the spirit of his times, a near inevitable failure born of the tension between persona and trickster dynamics, or all the above, is in some ways the lesser problem to work out. Our contemporary and pressing need is to create containers in which the dirt that trickster throws in our faces can serve as compost for the food that will feed future generations of Jungian analysts, those that come for analysis, and whatever we can provide for larger communities and culture. I hope that this book serves as one such container in which we continue the work of making the unfixed fixed, the fixed unfixed, dissolve and coagulate, and find the medicine in our afflictions.

If there has been a tacit agreement amongst us to not explore Jung's failures more openly, it is time to break that contract, open the crypts and explore the trauma in analytic communities. We now know that there are cultural and racialized *complexes* that are projected, and we also know that a phylogenetic image of the collective unconscious—often layered using a racial and misogynist bias—from primitive on upward, is not grounded in the reality of biology, neuroscience, or psychological development. Some of this knowledge is mortifying and some is liberating, and some of it brings up important questions that need exploration, such as whether, or not, the clinical method that arose from the image of a collective unconscious, archetypal amplification, bears traces of prior failure.

Africa makes a last appearance in Jung's final masterwork, *Mysterium Coniunctionis* (*MC;* 1963/1970). As one of the allegories for the individuation process in *MC*, Jung describes the imaginal journey of a medieval alchemist. The alchemist's journey comes to its end at the last of the four directions, 'south', in Africa, which Jung likened to the fourth function, the most heated and unconscious of all, in this case, interestingly, *intuition.* Satyrs, pans, dog-headed baboons, and "innumerable species of wild animals" (ibid., para 277) lived in this alchemical Africa. Another lived there as well: the Sibyl who foretold the coming of Christ. Mercurius was nearby, as was the mystical phoenix. Jung commented on these inhabitants and their activities:

In order to become the ever-living bird of the spirit, the alchemical animal soul needs the transforming fire which is found in 'Africa'. The mystery alluded to here is not only the encounter with the animal soul but, at the same time and in the same place, the meeting with the anima, a feminine psychopomp who showed him the way to Mercurius and also how to find the phoenix.

(ibid., para 282)

No longer fearing the transformative fire of the red-hot poker, Africa had finally become the heated cauldron in which the animal soul and the anima came together. Their liaison, and their encounter with the ancient alchemical trickster, was imagined to be the secret of resurrection and rebirth. Development. Gradual Progress.

Notes

1 For example, in the Grail legend, the naive young Parsifal comes upon the Grail Castle almost by chance but fails to ask crucial questions that would heal the Wasteland and the Fisher King's wound. This failure precipitates the immediate disappearance of the Grail Castle. Parsifal spends many years of searching the Wasteland for the Grail, and via the search, to finally understand its purpose (Johnson 1977).

   In Greek myth, Odysseus undergoes some epic failures. At the end of the journey his ships sink, all his men die, until he eventually makes it home, alone, an old man but whole.

   From another tradition, the African literature and oracular divination system of Ifa, (the god of time), is full of sad tales and fates of mythic characters who fail to grasp or perform the appropriate sacrifice indicated to them by the oracle (Bynum 1999).

2 A full discussion of the tension between pluralistic and unitary visions of psychological process (the myth of the Many and the One) held by the early founders of psychology can be found in Salman (2013).

3 Haeckel's recapitulation theory has been proven incorrect. For a full discussion see Gould (1981, 1985).

4 In the same passage Jung also opined that white Americans were infected by black Americans:

   The peculiar walk with loose joints, or the swinging of the hips so frequently observed in Americans, also comes from the Negro. American music draws its main inspiration from the Negro, and so does the dance. The expression of religious feeling, the revival meetings, the Holy Rollers, and other abnormalities are strongly influenced by the Negro, and the famous American naïveté, in its charming as well as its more unpleasant form, invites comparison with the childlikeness of the Negro. The vivacity of the average American, which shows itself not only at baseball games but quite particularly in his extraordinary love of talking—the ceaseless gabble of American papers is an eloquent example of this—is scarcely to be derived from his Germanic forefathers, but is far more like the chattering of a Negro village.

   (Jung 1927/1931, para 95)

5 Jung recounts being told that since whites were in Africa, dreams were no longer needed because the English already knew everything.

References

Abraham, N. & Torok, M. (1994). *The Shell and the Kernel: Renewals of psychoanalysis, Vol. 1*. Chicago: University of Chicago Press.

Burleson, B. (2005). 'The Wild Goose'. *Jung in Africa*. New York: Continuum.

Bynum, E.B. (1999). *The African Unconscious: Roots of ancient mysticism and modern psychology*. New York: Teacher's College Press.

Gould, S.J. (1981). *The Mismeasure of Man*. New York: W.W. Norton.

Gould, S.J. (1985). *Ontogeny and Phylogeny*. Cambridge: Harvard University Press.

Hyde, L. (1998). *Trickster Makes this World: How disruptive imagination creates culture*. New York: Canongate Books.

Johnson, R. (1977). *He: Understanding masculine psychology*. New York: Harper Collins.

Jung, C.G. (1917/1972). *Two Essays in Analytical Psychology, CW 7*.

Jung, C.G. (1927/1931). 'Mind and Earth', *CW 10*.

Jung, C.G. (1930/1964). 'The complications of American Psychology', *CW 10*.

Jung, C.G. (1931/1964). 'Archaic man', *CW 10*.

Jung, C.G. (1935/1976). 'The Tavistock Lectures: On the theory and practice of analytical psychology', *CW 18*.

Jung, C.G. (1939/1989). 'The Symbolic Life', *CW 18*.

Jung, C.G. (1946/1985). 'The psychology of the transference', *CW 16*.

Jung, C.G. (1948/1975). 'On the nature of dreams', *CW 8*.

Jung, C.G. (1953/1972). 'Negative attempts to free the individuality from the collective psyche', *CW 7*.

Jung, C.G. (1963/1970). *Mysterium Coniunctionis CW 14*.

Jung, C.G. (1963/1989). *Memories, Dreams, Reflections*. New York: Vintage Books.

Jung, C.G. (2009). *The Red Book. Liber Novus*. S. Shamdasani, ed. New York & London: W.W. Norton.

LaGamma, A. (2000). *Art and Oracle: African art and rituals of divination*. New York: Harry Abrams.

Machado, A. (1983). *Times Alone: Selected poems of Antonio Machado*. Middletown: Wesleyan University Press.

Reppen, J. & Schulman, M. (eds.) (2018). *Failures in Psychoanalytic Treatment*. New York: International Psychoanalytic Books.

Salman, S. (2006). 'True Imagination'. *Spring 47*. New Orleans: Spring: A journal of archetype and culture.

Salman, S. (2013). *Dreams of Totality: Where we are when there's nothing at the center*. New Orleans: Spring Journal Books, Inc.

Wilhelm, R. (ed. and trans.) (1950/1967). *The I Ching or Book of Changes*. New Jersey: Princeton University Press.

Winchester, S. (1998). *The Professor and the Madman: A tale of murder, insanity, and the making of the Oxford English Dictionary*. New York: Harper Collins.

Chapter 5

From Ghost to Ancestor
Transforming Jung's racial complex

Amy Bentley Lamborn

In a single poetic line, W. H. Auden expressed a truism that grounds and orients depth psychological theory. It is a truism that analysts witness both in their own lives and in virtually every analytic hour. Auden said that 'We are lived by powers we pretend to understand' (Auden 1939/1991). We may think we are in control of our lives—doing the right things, being "reasonable"—then something happens, and we are urged toward a reckoning: "Who is *really* in charge? Who or what lives behind and within the stories around which our lives unfold?" As James Hollis writes in his book, *Hauntings: Dispelling the Ghosts Who Run Our Lives,* 'we are inevitably impelled to witness that the present moment is informed by the past, driven by its imperatives, its prescriptions and proscriptions' (Hollis 2013/2015, p. xvi).

In this chapter, I shall lend understanding to two such powers: one that *lives us* in the manner of Auden's image (ghosts), and another that bequeaths to us *something worth living* (ancestors). What these powers have in common, of course, is their association with the realm of the dead, the underworld (Hillman 1979, p. 40). My interest is in the transformation of one of these powers (ghosts) into the other (ancestors), which presupposes a distinction between these two powers—a distinction that should not be collapsed. On this point, I agree with Samuel Kimbles who writes, 'The problem with that blurring of the distinction [between ghosts and ancestors] is that we may miss an opportunity to think about how we relate to and listen to the voices of our ancestors—or not' (Kimbles 2021, p. 26). This blurring of the distinction also means we miss an opportunity to think about how we relate (or not) to our ghosts, those 'spectral presences' that run our lives (Hollis 2013/2015).

What, then, is the distinction between ghosts and ancestors?

The etymology of ghost implies disembodied spirits which torment and terrify. Psychologically, ghosts are those complexes—whether personal or cultural—that have us in their grip. 'When we look at cultural complexes, for example, that come from trauma inflicted on one group by another', Ann Belford Ulanov writes, 'we see unfinished mourning, untransformed memories, wounded parts of self and community deposited in the children of the next generations' (Ulanov 2013, p. 46). Freud's famous formulation also comes to

DOI: 10.4324/9781003311447-6

mind: 'a thing which has not been understood inevitably reappears; like an unlaid ghost, it cannot rest until the mystery has been solved and the spell spoken' (Freud 1909, p. 123).

Ghosts haunt us with all that is unlived, unventured, unredeemed. Their phantom-like spectral presence often is felt as absence, which Kimbles calls an 'absent presence' (2021, p. 6). The 'phantomatic effects' of these ghosts are real; and they are visible, generation after generation. As Kimbles writes, '[These] intergenerational processes are expressed as phantoms that provide representation and continuity for unresolved or unworked-through grief and violence that occurred in a prior historical cultural context, providing for potential continuity of these dynamics' (2021, p. 12). Ghosts fuel our compulsion to repeat. The incapacities and failures of those who have gone before us live on in our current anxieties, attitudes, and entanglements.

The word *ancestor*, on the other hand, literally means 'to go before' (Lat. *antecedere*). An ancestor is a forefather, a predecessor, an antecedent. Ancestors live forth as vital lifeblood—flowing through us, connecting past to present, and reaching toward the future. Ancestors 'endow energy' as they pulsate in and through the rhythms of our lives (Ulanov 2013, p. 46). These shades of meaning are evident in James Hillman's definition of ancestors as 'the dead whose spirits continue to protect our work and urge it onward' (Hillman 2014, p. 231).

Psychologically, ancestors are complexes that have been worked-on and worked-through so that they are no longer split-off and siphoning away vital energy. Ancestors help us live zestfully and creatively. They bestow a sense of agency, generativity, and legacy. We witness such a bestowal in Bruce Springsteen's remarks during a conversation with Barak Obama, when each spoke about the legacies of their dead fathers. Springsteen said that we must turn our ghosts into ancestors. While ghosts haunt us, ancestors accompany us on our way; ancestors offer us comfort and give us a perspective on life that we make our own. Springsteen said that his father now walks with him as his ancestor. But that transformation—from ghost to ancestor—was a long time in the making (*The Guardian*, 3 October 2021).

It has been a long time since Carl Gustav Jung's death—more than fifty years, in fact; but his ghost remains very much alive. Recent accounts of Jung's life and work have laid out more problematic aspects of Jung's writings, especially in relation to his use of such terms as 'Aryan', 'Jewish', and 'primitive'. Carrie Dohe's *Jung's Wandering Archetype: Race and Religion in Analytical Psychology* is one such account. Dohe argues that Jung used science to give cover to dangerous racial stereotypes that were of common use in early twentieth-century Europe, stereotypes that are being used dangerously yet today (Dohe 2016). Some turn a blind eye to Jung's ghost. Others seek to rationalize it. Still others think it needs to be exorcised, driven out, expelled. Instead of ignoring, excusing, or expunging Jung's ghost, I am holding out for the possibility of its transformation by participating in what psychoanalyst Sam Gerson describes as 'the creative act of altering the hauntings of the past into a base from which development may proceed—and so ... partake in the project [Hans] Loewald (1980) so aptly described as the movement of ghost into ancestors' (2016, p. 203).

Is not the way of transformation what Jung, himself, depicted for us?

Ghosts: a *Red Book* encounter

Of the many provocative scenes in *The Red Book*, one stands out for its vivid imagining of ghosts. In the "Divine Folly", Jung finds himself in the anteroom of a large hall with high ceilings and green curtains (Jung 2009, p. 328). After discovering one room after another, Jung sees two doors on a rear wall. He enters the door on the right, upon which he discovers the reading room of a vast library. When the librarian inquires about Jung's reading interests, Jung unthinkingly requests a copy of Thomas à Kempis's *The Imitation of Christ*. Jung's choice prompts a dialogue with the librarian, who wonders what philosophical, theological, or prayerful interest Jung might have in this rarely sought-after text (ibid., p. 320).

After receiving the book and having a spirited conversation with the librarian, Jung departs the reading room while contemplating the true meaning of the *imitatio Christi*. 'If I thus truly imitate Christ, I do not imitate anyone, I emulate no one, but go my own way ... ' (Jung 2009, p. 232). Jung soon finds himself standing again in the anteroom, where he again sees the door on the left. Like the door to the right, it remains open. Jung enters this door, which opens to a spacious kitchen. There is a large chimney above the stove. There are two long tables in the middle of the room, surrounded by benches. There are brass and copper pots and all kinds of cooking vessels on the shelves. A large woman, presumably the cook, is standing at the stove. Jung asks her if he might sit while he waits for something to happen (ibid., p. 333).

Jung takes his book from his pocket and begins to read. The cook notices the title and wonders whether Jung was a cleric. She tells Jung that her mother had owned *The Imitation of Christ*. It had been special to her mother, who had the book with her on her deathbed, and she had given it to the cook before she died. While the cook is still speaking, Jung begins to browse through the book. Immersed in his thoughts, Jung admits his desire to imitate Christ. Just then, Jung is seized by 'an inner disquiet' and wonders what is happening: 'I hear an odd swishing and whirring—and suddenly a roaring sound fills the room like a horde of large birds—with a frenzied flapping of wings—I see many shadow-like human forms rush past and I hear a manifold babble of voices utter the words: "Let us pray in the temple"' (Jung 2009, p. 334).

Jung speaks to this manifold babble of voices, asking it where it is 'rushing off to' (Jung 2009, p. 334). At that point 'a bearded man with tousled hair and dark shining eyes stops and turns toward me: "We are wandering to Jerusalem to pray at the most holy sepulcher"' (ibid., p.335). Jung asks the man to take him with them to Jerusalem. But the man tells Jung that he cannot join them because he has a body. *They* are dead—Ezekiel, an Anabaptist, and a whole throng of fellow believers. They cannot stop wandering because they must make a pilgrimage to all the holy places. They are driven to wander because, although they died in 'true belief', they 'still have no peace', for they had not come to a proper end with their lives. 'It seems to me that we forgot something important that should also be lived' (ibid.).

Jung presses to know what this important, unlived thing was. The man asks in turn, 'Would you happen to know?' With these words the man 'reaches out greedily and uncannily' toward Jung, 'his eyes shining as if from inner heat'. Jung shouts, 'Let go, daimon, you did not live your animal' (Jung 2009, p. 335).[1]

The cook is horrified by Jung's encounter with this multitude of the dead: 'For God's sake ... . Help, what's wrong with you?' (Jung 2009, p. 336). Strange people soon burst into the room, 'infinitely astonished and dismayed at first, then laughing maliciously: "Oh, I might have known, exclaims the librarian. Quick, the police"'. Jung is dragged off to the madhouse, where he is diagnosed with 'a form of religious madness ... religious paranoia'. Jung is interviewed, undressed, bathed, then taken to the ward before being put to bed. There he contemplates his 'divine madness' (ibid., pp. 336–38).[2]

Jung realizes that the 'imitation of Christ' had led him to Christ's kingdom (Jung 2009, p. 339). There the '"mercy of God" signifies a particular/state of the soul' in which he must give himself 'to all neighbors with trembling and hesitation and with the mightiest outlay of hope that everything will work out well' (ibid.). Jung feels 'a shivering horror' that he has 'fallen into the boundless, the abyss, the inanity of eternal chaos', which rushes towards him 'as if carried by the roaring wings of a storm, the hurtling waves of the sea'. This chaos is 'an unending multiplicity,' filled with confusing and over-whelming figures (ibid., pp. 339–40).

Who are these figures? Who are those who rushed past Jung on their way to Jerusalem? In the madhouse, deeply immersed in his feelings, Jung gains an understanding of the identities of the dead:

These figures are the dead, not just your dead, that is, all the images of the shapes you took in the past, which your ongoing life has left behind, but also the thronging dead of human history, the ghostly procession of the past, which is an ocean compared to the drops of your own life span. I see behind you, behind the mirror of your eyes, the crush of dangerous shadows, the dead, who look greedily through the empty sockets of your eyes, who moan and hope to gather up through you all the loose ends of the ages, which sigh in them. ... Put your ear to that wall and you will hear the rustling of their procession ... . What you excluded from your life, what you renounced and damned, everything that was and could have gone wrong, awaits you behind that wall before which you sit quietly.

(Jung 2009, p. 340)

These figures arise like 'ghostly remainders' from the margins, 'sniping from the sidelines and the depths; harrying us as we go about our lives' (Frosh 2013, p. 3). As *The Red Book* makes clear, it is not just our personal dead who haunt us. The collective weight of human history is 'the ghostly procession of the past'.

Dwelling with the shades: *anamnesis*

In *Hauntings: Psychoanalysis and Ghostly Transmissions,* Stephen Frosh observes:

> To be haunted is … to be influenced by a kind of inner voice that will not stop speaking and cannot be excised, that keeps cropping up to trouble us and stop us going peaceably on our way. It is to harbour a presence that we are aware of, sometimes overwhelmed by, that embodies elements of past experience and future anxiety and hope, and that will not let us be.
> (Frosh 2013, pp. 2–3)

In 'The Divine Folly', we witness ghosts from the past who overwhelm Jung and will not let him be. His encounters with these ghosts attest to the porous line between the living and the dead. Indeed, throughout *The Red Book*, Jung comes face-to-face with death's 'imminence'—the reality that '*In the midst of life, we are in death*' (Hillman & Shamdasani 2013, p. 84; *italics mine*). In Jung's fantasy, the dead are *there,* just behind the wall. With his ear to the wall, Jung hears the rustling and frenzied flapping of their bird-like procession. Jung must learn 'to dwell among the shades … to be present in and among what is already here but not in a tangible, visible way' (Jung 2009, p. 226).

Dwelling with the shades requires an active, often frightening engagement with that which haunts and snips at us from the margins of our awareness. *The Red Book* is filled with such terrifying encounters. 'The dead want to take you over', Hillman writes. 'It is … a quite literal possession that is at play there' (Hillman and Shamdasani 2013, p. 26). In the madhouse, Jung sits quietly on one side of the wall, while the dead await on the other side, moaning with all that is unfinished, excluded, renounced, with 'the crush of dangerous shadows' (Jung 2009, p. 340).

By dwelling with the shades, Jung becomes the hero of *The Red Book's* epic saga. The restoration of the dead, the individuation of the dead, is part of Jung's heroic task. That is what the *Imitation of Christ* revealed to Jung—'the love Christ had for the widest range of human persons, including the lowest and highest qualities and impulses in each individual' (Slattery 2011, p. 136).

Bringing together the highest and lowest is fundamentally the work of remembrance. As Hillman explains:

> It's the opening to the dead and the deeply personal. And the deeply personal is connecting back through history, it's connecting to all that's been left out and forgotten … . The process is one of connection or restoration or remembrance … . The process of remembering. Anamnesis.
>
> (Hillman & Shamdasani 2013, p. 96)

Anamnesis is the opposite of amnesia. It implies a *re*-membering, a *re*-collection. As such, anamnesis is concerned with the *fullness* of memory, including dismissed and forgotten elements of human experiences. *Anamnesis* is a bringing of the past into the present so that a process of integration can commence. Sonu Shamdasani thus admonishes:

> The questions of the living, the problems of the living, the suffering of the living can be answered, or addressed, only through attending to the dead … Unless you manage to situate yourself with regard to the dead, you can't find a solution to your own living.
>
> (ibid., p.175)

What, then, does it mean to dwell with Jung's shade? How do we situate ourselves regarding Jung's life, with its flaws and imperfections? What left-out, ignored, and distorted dimensions of Jung's own life and work need to be gathered, re-collected, re-membered? And especially in the context of these reflections, how do we relate to Jung's racial complex?

Christopher J. Carter has recently asserted that many of Jung's writings 'are soiled with pejorative declarations that add nothing to analytic theory, but belittle, demean, and propagandize against non-Europeans, with a special intolerance toward African Americans' (2021, p. 74). His is a stinging critique. But we must reckon with the fact that Jung's racial complex is on display throughout the *Collected Works* as well as in *Memories Dreams and Reflections* (1961/2011). It is also evident in accounts of Jung's teaching and his training of the first generation of analysts. In the *Visions Seminars*, for example, Jung said:

> It is quite astonishing to see how little the primitive can actively think. He cannot concentrate, he has no power of attention. If the thing doesn't catch his instinct, he is as if unaware; that is, he has a passive awareness, but it doesn't move him in the least.
>
> (Jung 1997, p. 210)

The examples Jung gives of 'primitivity' here include a ritual of the 'Australian Negroes' and a 'famous story' about a sick 'nigger' (Jung 1997, pp. 210–11). Worse, Jung's thinking about primitivity is often linked with his theoretical concepts and formulations. As Helen Morgan puts it, 'Jung was quite emphatic about the psyche of the "primitive" as he was about the danger for the white man of "going black" through contamination, and he linked much of his pronouncements to the collective unconscious' (Morgan 2004, p. 219).[3]

In her Introduction to the *Visions Seminars*, Claire Douglas reflects on the attitudes and biases Jung displayed in the seminar from the vantage point of the late twentieth-century. In her assessment of Jung's treatment of his analysand Christiana Morgan (the focus of the seminar), Douglas writes that Jung had seemingly 'reached the limits of his era's masculine understanding of the feminine' and that this place of limitation allowed 'the shadow side of Jung's explorer stance to break through in the raw' (Douglas 1997, p. xxvi). Douglas recalls Jung treating Morgan 'as an alien, more primitive, *other*, in the same unconsciously patronizing way that male explorers of Jung's era tended to treat any gender, race, religion, or culture different from their own' (ibid.). Douglas describes and assesses this raw breakthrough of Jung's shadow in two sentences:

> Where this is played out in the seminar is in a few problematical word usages and tall tales that today, in the English-speaking world, would be labeled racist. They mar the seminar whether they stem from Jung's delight in American slang (and perhaps a language problem) that caused him to equate the words 'nigger' and 'Negro' or from the white man's bias so prevalent in the anthropological sources then available to him.
>
> (Douglas 1997, p. xxvi)

Douglas describes the edges of Jung's shadow, admitting that his racial complex tarnished the seminar. But she also attempts to soften the impact of Jung's language and behavior by minimizing it, offering counterexamples, and sharing one of Jung's prescient observations:

> When [Jung] deals with particulars and particular individuals, as in his religious discussions with the black headman during his 1925–31 African Safari, Jung is related, respectful, and astute. At times in the seminar he seems to free himself from the common projection on African society: "We suffer from the inflation of the white man, but naturally the inflation will be pricked and we shall collapse.
>
> (Douglas 1997, p. xxvi)

Douglas ultimately excuses Jung's biased thinking and racist rhetoric, invoking the limitations of his historical-cultural standpoint, lauding his marvel at the psyche, and identifying the ease with which he could self-correct:

Jung should not be blamed for falling into this trap; no one can view his or her own time and culture from a place outside its confines. Consciously and at his best, Jung was filled with awed wonder at the psyche in all its forms and as able to correct his biases rapidly when he found someone sufficiently secure to enlighten him. The seminar members could not, as they were caught in the same historical moment as well as their roles as students and analysands.

(Douglas 1997, pp. xxvi–xxvii)

Carter states that the 'man of his time' excuse for 'Jung's mercurial applications of *primitive* is 'lackluster' ... 'hollow' (2021, p. 72). Everyone is 'deeply influenced by time', Carter maintains; 'there remains a wide spectrum of attitudes and choices' (ibid.). Margorie Florestal, for example, invokes the abolitionists, the freedom fighters, the leaders of the Civil Rights movement—all men and women who were also people of their times. 'History is replete with examples of those who refused to project cultural shadow on the maligned groups of their era', Florestal writes. Additionally, she recalls that Jung's contemporary, the British psychoanalyst D. W. Winnicott, criticized his government's silence regarding the Nazis (Florestal 2014, p. 6).

Still, 'the spirit of the times ... coloured Jung's attitudes and projections towards persons with African ancestry' (Vaughan 2019, p. 322). To be sure, the limitations of Jung's historical-cultural context, cannot simply be ignored. Yet when 'historical context' is used to minimize responsibility rather than to contextualize socio-cultural influences, it amounts to a whitewashing of Jung and analytic theory. According to Merriam-Webster, the meaning of *whitewash* is:

To gloss over or cover up; to exonerate; to hold (an opponent) scoreless in a game; to alter in a way that favors, features, or caters to white people (such as to portray the past in a way that increases the prominence, relevance, or impact of white people and minimizes or misrepresents that of nonwhite people).

(Brown 2020)

There is a fine line between offering an historical perspective and laboring to exonerate. When the 'Jung was a man of his time' response is used to whitewash, the 'offence adheres' (Carter 2021, p. 72).

In *The Work of Whiteness*, Helen Morgan identifies whitewashing as an example of the 'disavowal of whiteness', which she sees as the typical racism of white liberals. The disavowal of whiteness, in contrast to white supremacy, is a psychological defense operating 'at the more invisible level of white privilege and white solipsism' (Morgan 2021, p. 3). To explain this defense, Morgan invokes the concept of psychological splitting, especially Heinz Kohut's notion of the vertical split within the structure of the ego:

I suggest this vertical split as it relates to racism is not merely a single line dividing two parts of the psyche, with the investment in white privilege and the racist thought on one side, and the condemnation and rejection of racism in the other side. On both sides there remains a capacity for symbolization which is lacking in certain moments when we are reminded of our racism. The internal psychic structure can be imagined as made up of two vertical layers between which there is a gap, a silent, empty place devoid of symbols in which it is impossible to play or grieve.

(Morgan 2021, p. 67)

Morgan contends that this silent and empty gap, devoid of symbols, is a kind of '*psychose blanche*' (ibid., pp. 66–67). Quoting Adrianne Harris:

It may be that there is in "whiteness" a "psychose blanche" named by André Green (1970) for quite other purposes. Deeper than depression, deeper than rage, there is a blankness, a place where there is not sufficient structure for mourning, where the psyche gives way. Perhaps this is what "whiteness" is: the disruption or erasure of mourning, a gap in the psyche, which through "whiteness" functions like an imploding star, refusing signification. It is not trauma solely that is whitened out but also destructiveness and memory.[4]

(Morgan 2021, p. 67)

Outright silence about racism is another manifestation of *psychose blanche*, and there exists a deafening silence about Jung's racism in the Jungian world. In an "Open Letter from a group of Jungians on the questions of Jung's writing on and theories about 'Africans'" (2019), Jungians scholars, clinicians, and analysts from around the world called for an end to this silence. The letter specifically references the thirty years since the publication of Farhad Dalal's 'Jung: A racist' (1988), after which neither an acknowledgement nor an apology was forthcoming:

Analytical psychologists and other Jungians have known about the implications of Jung's ideas for decades; there are signatories to this Letter who have campaigned for recognition of the problems. But there has been a failure to address them responsibly, seriously and in public.

(Open Letter, p. 361)

The signatories are clear and forthright about the implications of Jung's racial ideology:

We share the concern that Jung's colonial and racist ideas – sometimes explicit and sometimes implied – have led to inner harm (for example, internalized inferiority and self-abnegation) and outer harm (such as interpersonal and social consequences) for the groups, communities and individuals mentioned ... . Moreover, in the opinion of the signatories to this letter, these ideas have also led to aspects of *de facto* institutional and structural racism being present in Jungian organizations.

(Open Letter, p. 361)

Psychose blanche causes both internal and external suffering. Its 'imploding star'-like dynamic can render us speechless, even hopeless. Yet, '*The suffering of the living can only be answered through attending to the dead*' (Hillman & Shamdasani, p. 175). Dwelling with the shades is how we begin to heal *psychose blanche*, that maddening gap in which "whiteness" itself disrupts mourning for what is lost and erases the awareness of our capacity for destructiveness and our memory of what has happened and of what we have done. Jung's racial complex is real, as is its harm to individuals and groups. It continues to injure both non-whites and whites alike. Still, we must remember that, as with all complexes, the racial complex holds the potential of being transformed from a ghost that haunts to an ancestor who walks with us, urging us onward in our life and work. In her extended reflection on *The Red Book,* Ann Ulanov describes it this way:

> Despite our fear that our complex makes us mad forever, imprisoning us in sterile rigidity or scattering us into chaotic fragments, in facing it our descent can turn into quest for redemptive force. We long for another way of seeing so that what falls apart may re-form into new wholes with different levels of meaning. In that nowhere place of disruption that our complex causes, we can speak of homelessness, contingency, irretrievable losses. We see the cost of our complex: ruined relationships, others hurt, spoiled opportunities. From such grief we yearn for integration. Our complex forces a path, speaking for completeness, bringing what is left out, impelling us to integrate our wholeness.
>
> (Ulanov 2013, p. 56)

Both our personal complexes and our cultural complexes can be transformed into 'creative legacies' through which our psychic splits are healed and through which 'nowhere' gaps become spaces 'for the unbearable and for what is not yet here' (ibid., pp. 67). I use the ancient term *chora* (Gr. Χώρα: "country", "land") to depict such a space.[5]

In the *Timeaus* dialogue, Plato invoked *chora* to account for his "third thing" between Forms and Copies. He used a variety of images to capture *chora*'s elusive nature, including mother, womb, receptacle, nurse, space, a base material for the making of perfume, a land region, and a winnowing sieve used in the bread-making process (Plato 1997, p. 1255). Chora thus links associatively with the kitchen scene from *The Red Book* and the 'realm of the mothers', the place in which Jung encounters the dead in 'The Divine Folly'.[6]

In more contemporary imaginings, chora is sometimes identified as a yawning gap-like space; a no-place, abyssal and empty. Such is the space Jung experiences when he feels that he has 'fallen into the boundless, the abyss, the inanity of eternal chaos' (Jung 2009, p. 339).

The verb form of chora (*chorien*: "to make room for", "to contain") suggests an additional interpretative trajectory. Byzantine artwork such as that which is found in the Chora Church (Istanbul) affirms this alternative possibility. Rather than invoking a boundless, chaotic, abyssal emptiness, this artwork images chora as aliveness and as boundless containment. A mural of Christ is inscribed with *Khôra of all the Living*. A mural depicting Mary, Mother of God holding the Christ-child is inscribed with the phrase '*khora tou akhoretou*', *Container of the Uncontainable*. These inscriptions amplify that which the *Imitation of Christ* reveals to Jung in 'The Divine Folly': 'the love Christ had for the widest range of human persons, including the lowest and highest qualities and impulses in each individual' (Slattery 2011, p. 136).

The abyssal, gap-like chora—where the psyche gives way and memory is threatened with erasure—becomes a space of *anamnesis* in which all that has been disavowed, excluded, or damned can be gathered. It becomes a space in which Jung's ghost can be held and transformed. Chora is a generative space in which Jung's 'divine madness', and our own, might dwell and heal (Kearney 2003, p. 194).

Ancestor: the *opus contra naturum*

I have considered 'dwelling with the shades' as it pertains to ghosts and their hauntings. In this section, I will invoke another meaning of *shade,* the one having to do with color ... particularly *alchemical color*. As James Hillman reminds us, 'alchemical colors are in the world, of the world, and tell us about the world' (1986, p. 44). Here, we shall traverse a path through whiteness, its shadows, and eventually its shades. Specifically, I will reflect on an archetypal-psychological approach that Hillman offers as a structural therapy of racism, which he painstakingly outlines in "Notes on White Supremacy" (ibid., p. 29).[7]

In reviewing Hillman's line of thinking, I will demonstrate that his archetypal psychologizing gives us a path toward a more profound healing of *psychose blanche*. I will also show that his understanding of alchemy's struggle against whiteness offers an archetypal perspective on the kind of *anamnesis* necessary for the transformation of ghosts into ancestors. As Hillman observes, there is a kind of white that 'remembers its forebears, its drop of black blood, blue blood. Its whiteness is the complete presence of all hues, not their absence, including hues yet to be born' (Hillman 1986, p. 51). This 'psychological white', the white that has an *anamnesis* of its forebears, is born of alchemy's opus—an *opus contra naturum*—in which whiteness, along with all alchemical colors, is transmuted.

Context and aims

Hillman's thesis is clear from the outset: *the fantasy of white supremacy is archetypally rooted and structured; and this supremacy is inherent in the very concept of whiteness.* By archetypal, he means 'geographically distributed, temporally enduring, and emotionally charged'. Hillman aims to differentiate this intrinsic archetypal structure, thereby offering a way 'of ameliorating the archetypal curse of supremacy beyond the usual and necessary societal measures' (1986, pp. 29–30). Note that Hillman does not advocate that we forego socio-cultural methods to deal with white supremacy. He rather offers a distinctly psychological method—symbolic and interpretive—*in addition to* these other critical modes of engagement.

Hillman sees himself approaching the root of the problem: our culture is white supremacist and the 'superiority of whiteness' is reinforced both by our written texts and in our linguistic foundations. In sum, 'we tend to see white as first, as best, as most embracing,' Hillman writes, 'and define it in superior terms' (1986, p. 29).

Hillman cites a range of evidence, including anthropological, historical, and mythological, to argue that 'whiteness has had archetypal supremacy over blackness in the psyches of both whites and blacks' (Adams 1996, p. 26). For example, he considers the anthropologist Victor Turner's research into the color classifications of the Ndembu of Zambia, whose definition of "white" includes 'goodness, strength, purity, free of misfortune, of death, of sorrow, of ridicule … to sweep clean, wash … .' For the Ndembu:

> whiteness, more than any color, represents the divinity as essence and source, as well as sustentation. White as light streaming forth from the divinity has … a quality of trustworthiness and veracity … . White is also unsullied and unpolluted … . Behind the symbolism of whiteness, then, lie the notions of harmony, continuity, purity, the manifest, the public, the appropriate, and the legitimate.
>
> (Hillman 1986, p. 32)

From the archetypal perspective, we are all white supremacists (Adams 1996, p. 24).

Whiteness: three clusters of archetypal meaning

Informed by etymological and linguistic studies, Hillman distinguishes three main meanings of white and considers each as if it were a perspective governed by a particular archetype: (1) *heavenly/spiritual white*—the white of divinity, which has to do with purity and sanctity; (2) *the white of innocence,* commonly associated with the archetypal child, without corruption, pollution, illness, evil; and (3) *anima white*—connected with the female/feminine (i.e., the "white goddess"), as well as vulnerability and effeminacy. Again, Hillman does not intend to reify the semantics of whiteness, but rather to differentiate it from these archetypal resonances.[8] 'Each white bears its specific triumph and specific threat together', he writes, 'that is, each white offers one of the supremacies together with the shadow specific to that supremacy' (Hillman 1986, p. 41).

The problem beneath the supremacy of white is that we perceive whiteness and blackness as opposites rather than acknowledging the differences between them. As Michael Vannoy Adams puts it, 'white is a color that presumes that it is never wrong but always right ... ; it is a light that shines so bright that it blinds the eye—obliterates all differences, all other shadows, all other shades of color' (Adams 1996, p. 27). The work of differentiation, however, gives us another way of seeing. 'Differences neither compete, contradict nor oppose', Hillman writes. 'To be different as night and day does not require an opposition of night and day' (Hillman 1986, p. 39).

The white unconscious

Without differentiation, Hillman concludes, 'white casts its own white shadow', or better, that '*white sees its own shadow in black*' (1986, p. 41; *italics mine*). Seeing white "here" while simultaneously seeing black "over there" is the essence of shadow projection. 'This psychological rule,' Hillman writes, 'became the historical case' (ibid.). The *Oxford English Dictionary* reports that the first use of the word *white* to describe an ethnic group occurred in 1604, following the perception of African people as *black*. Oppositional thinking, thinking in black-and-white, was there at the beginning:

> Peoples identified *by* color became identified *with* color; Africans who did not perceive themselves as "blacks" became "blacks," a discovery of the white unconscious. West African society begins psychologically not in the structures of black society ... nor even in the inherent supremacy of whiteness described above ... but rather in oppositional thinking.
>
> (Hillman 1986, p. 42)

This 'blackening' already resided inside the word *black* well before any English-speaking explorer arrived on the shores of West Africa. The *OED* tells us that, before the sixteenth century, the meaning of black included: 'Deeply stained with dirt; soiled, dirty, foul ... . Having dark or deadly purposes, malignant; pertaining to death, deadly; baneful, sinister ... . Foul, iniquitous, atrocious, horrible, wicked ... . Indicating disgrace, censure, liability to punishment, etc.'. Hillman argues:

> A logic of opposites preserves these foul notions. White would have no deadly purposes, could not be iniquitous and wicked or liable to punishment.

White folk are clean and censure-free, as if white ethnic identity was itself a baptismal font assuring salvation, as if alone the language of white by virtue of its archetypal resonances could restore purity, eliminate sin and guilt and shame.

(Hillman 1986, p. 43)

It is not my aim to provide a full historical account of the social construction of race. Nor am I attempting to summarize fully Hillman's account. What I intend to relate is this critical understanding: *that the sixteenth century geographical discoveries, with their concurrent deployment of the terms "whiteness" and "blackness" to categorize ethnic identities, coincided with seeing Africa through the lens of white consciousness. And this way of seeing "Africa" informed what became the geography of psyche.* 'The topological language used by Freud for "the unconscious" as a place below, different, timeless, primordial, libidinal and separated from consciousness recapitulates what white reporters centuries earlier said about West Africa' (Hillman 1986, p. 45).

Part of psychology's myth is that the unconscious was 'discovered' as its contents were 'explored'. Moreover, the idea that the unconscious was a "discovery" of something distinct from consciousness maintains the same white unconsciousness that 'consciousness' was formulated to challenge. Hillman asserts that 'it is this unconscious white consciousness that is the proper object of depth psychology, depth psychology come home to roost, out of Africa' (1986, pp. 44–45). So, while Hillman insists on the importance of Jung's notion of *shadow*, with its manifestation of depth and its reminder to withdraw projections, he also interrogates the term and concludes that shadow is, itself, compromised by its unconsciousness:

Though serving the aim of self-correction, the ideas of shadow and unconscious maintain the theory of opposites and locate consciousness with light, day, bright, active, etc. And so the entire modern psychological effort to raise consciousness, and the ego drafted to enact the endeavor, is one more manifestation of whiteness, perpetuating the very fault it would resolve.

(Hillman 1986, p. 47)

In his analysis of Hillman's 'Notes', Adams concludes that to address the problem of white supremacy effectively, we need to 'imagine differentially rather than oppositionally' (Adams 1997, p. 27). This differential imagination will find its bearings not in the modernist referential paradigm (which 'assumed that consciousness referred to "something literal, opaque, outside itself"'), but rather in a post-modernist, reflexive one. 'Instead of referring to objects in the external world, we will all, white and black, need to reflect further on ourselves—and on whiteness itself' (ibid.). Hillman's proposal for solving the problem of racism, Adams observes, 'requires reflection and imagination—or reimagination'. He argues that 'a psychoanalysis that would effectively challenge the supremacy of whiteness, the supremacy of consciousness, would eschew the white–black, conscious–unconscious oppositions ... and, instead, emphasize differences in degree rather than kind. It would accentuate the nuances' (Adams 1996, p. 28).

Alchemy and the world

Hillman turns to alchemy for such a differential imagining. Recalling Jung's turn to alchemy in the latter part of his life (which was, for Jung, a *return* to a color—both a 'colored soul and a colored world'), Hillman claims that Jung made another kind of return:

> It was also a return to that bifurcation in psychological history exemplified in the seventeenth century when white assumed its supremacy in science, geography, anthropology, and moral philosophy, and when colonialism, black slavery, the Enlightenment and Protestant monotheism were emerging as dominants in northern-western consciousness.
>
> (Hillman 1986, p. 49)

Alchemy reopens these social-historical issues, 'offering both penetration to their archetypal depths and the possibility of their transmutation' (Hillman 1986, p. 49). It self-corrects the interrelated ideas Hillman explores in his 'Notes', namely, 'repression and projection, oppositional thinking or splitting, superiority, invulnerability ... heaven-sent surety'—attitudes archetypally inherent in white's supremacy' (ibid.). As we shall see, alchemy's appreciation of color 'recognizes shadows within any hue', thus presenting us with an altogether different perspective on the supremacy of white. Hillman observes:

> Because its work is called an *opus contra naturam*, it sees (and hears) through what comes naturally, first, and easily to mind. Heavenly white, innocent white and anima calmness are all too simple. The *opus contra naturam* sophisticates its own fundamentals—its elements, its metals and heat.
>
> (Hillman 1986, p. 49)

Heavenly white, innocent white, anima white ... each of these clusters of meaning appear within the alchemical process. Hillman calls to mind the white names alchemy gives to the *prima materia*: white moisture, white smoke, the Bride/Eve, the Virgin's milk, cleansing Lye, Spring, Moon, the Lamb—whether heavenly/divine, shining, pure/purifying, innocent, or feminine. And the vulnerable white finds its adjunct in the whitening (*albedo*) process in alchemy. This anima whiteness is "superior", not in a heavenly or spiritual sense, but rather more in its effects. 'For the experience of the psyche's whitening is usually one of comforting ease', Hillman explains, 'a lifting of the burdensome nigredo where all was occluded' (Hillman 1986, pp. 36–37). The *albedo* softens the mood and lightens the atmosphere. 'Now one rests content on the moon', writes Hillman, 'supreme in one's lustrated psychological distance, Luna the Queen, all conflicting hues faded into the equanimity of white ... ' (ibid.).

Jung observed that for many alchemists the *albedo* was the climax of the work, the stage where 'all becomes one' (Jung 1963/1989, para. 388). This oneness, according to Hillman, is the 'smooth white notion of wholeness'— a 'lunar unity' (Hillman 1986, p. 37). But the process does not stop with the *albedo*. Instead, one is plunged back into the dreamy, innocent ignorant first thing—back into the *prima materia*. So, again we increase the heat toward yellow and red. We move back down and around again (*circulatio*). We repeat, yet again (*iteratio*) (ibid., p. 38).

Alchemy's iterative *circulatio* thus gives us another meaning of the 'work of whiteness,' for alchemy is 'a work against whiteness even as it strives to attain whiteness' (Hillman 1986, p. 50). *Opus contra naturum*—seeing and hearing through the things which come to mind first, naturally, and easily (ibid., p. 49). 'For the true alchemical white bears blackness within it, the blues of memory and regret, as it intends toward a further dawning, a waking-up to itself by yellowing. It is not sheer white, mere white, in fact, *no longer purely white at all*' (ibid., pp. 37–38). This psychological white results from the *nigredo*. Now psychologically stained and shaded, it is no longer innocent. 'Alchemy describes the breakdown of the white mind as the nigredo prior to and inherent within another white' (ibid., p. 51). The healing of *psychose blanche* requires this kind of breakdown—this kind of *anamnesis*—for this psychological white '*remembers its forebears, its drop of black blood, blue blood. Its whiteness is the complete presence of all things, not their absence, including hues yet to be born*'.

We dwell, also, with these shades.

Loving Jung

Together, these reflections have opened onto a question: 'How do I love Jung?' My love for Jung has never been in question, but the way I love Jung has shifted over time.

Now my manner of loving Jung is, itself, an *opus contra naturum*. It is a work with no hint of self-blinding idealization, no splitting off the bad, no projection of invulnerability onto Jung's life or work. My way of loving Jung bears the blackness of *nigredo*, the blues of anamnesis. Dwelling with Jung's shade, my forebearer is re-membered, re-collected. Claiming him as my ancestor with this kind of love frees up vital energy for thinking Jung forward in the present generation.

Jung's soul speaks of this manner of loving in *The Black Books*. As Jung struggled with his inner solitude and the horrible chaos over which he felt powerless—as he encountered the formless, abyssal chora, in which there are no 'straight lines or solid points'—he asked his soul how he could create order: 'Shall I begin with the nearest?' Soul replies, 'Or maybe with the furthest. To do the nearest is good for beginners' (Jung 2020, p. 207). *Opus contra naturum*. Jung's soul admonishes him to see through that which comes first, or naturally, or with ease. 'What is the furthest?' Jung asks. Soul offers a mysterious reply: 'Love inside out' (ibid.). What absolute craziness! How is Jung to understand this way of loving? Soul explains:

> There is straightforward love and love inside-out … . Straightforward love [is] direct love. Love inside-out is better described as indirect love. To my way of thinking loving someone indirectly is to love their obverse. Love the generosity of the miser, the ugly of the beautiful, the rationality of the crazy and the badness of the good.
>
> (Jung 2020, p. 207)

'That's asking for a lot', Jung replies. 'I doubt that I can do it. Might I begin with myself?' Soul says that one must always begin with oneself, by looking at oneself 'in the mirrors of others' (ibid.). It *is* asking for a lot, this crazy, inside-out way of loving. But Jung's soul insists that loving inside-out is how we realize 'the inner identity of the opposites' (Jung 2020, p. 207). Inside-out love is an alchemical love which overcomes all gaps, all splits, all oppositions. As the alchemical saying goes, *as within, so without*. 'The alchemical opus takes place *in vitro* and *in vivo*. There is the vessel of the world which too is psyche' (Hillman 1986, p. 52).

Loving Jung inside-out thus matters in and for the world. Jung's theory continues to hold up a mirror for me. And, in claiming Jung as an ancestor, I hold up a mirror for him, from my own time and place, with its own limitations and challenges … its own yearning for the depths. Loving Jung inside-out makes space 'for the unbearable and for what is not yet here'. Loving Jung inside-out takes place in the chora of the world, the container of the uncontainable. Loving Jung inside-out transforms the ghost that haunts us to an ancestor who urges us onward, bequeathing to us a creative legacy.

What hues may yet be born?

Notes

1   As *The Red Book* notes, in 1918 Jung had claimed that Christianity had 'suppressed the animal element', leaving out the instinctual (see "The Role of the Unconscious", CW 10, para. 31).
2   Of divine madness, Jung writes that it is 'a higher form of the irrationality of the life streaming through us … a madness that cannot be integrated into present-day society' (2009, p. 338).
3   Michael Vannoy Adams (1996) notes:

> In the colonialist, imperialist context, to go black was to revert—or, in psychoanalytic terms, to regress—to an earlier or lower state … . To go black is to "go back"—in time and space. This reversion is a regression not … in the "service of the ego" but, rather, in the service of the id, or instinct. To go black is

to "go instinctive". It is to return to a before and a beneath, to a state or state that the civilized white European, whether British or not, has presumably superseded.
(pp. 51–52)

4 Morgan further writes, 'Green's concept, 'psychose blanche', refers to a hole in the psyche created by the child's experience of the *dead mother*. As Green points out, this does not relate to the situation where the mother has died, but one where her previously lively engagement with the child is interrupted following an experience of loss—such as through a bereavement or a miscarriage. The term 'blanche' in French can mean either "white" or "blank" and Green uses it to refer to a problem of emptiness, or a negative that follows a decathexis of the maternal object. Mourning cannot take place, nor can the loss be symbolized' (2021, p. 67).

5 For an example, see Amy Bentley Lamborn's 'The Deus Absconditus and the Post-Secular Quest' (2014, pp. 203–13).

6 Symbolically, the setting of the kitchen, as a place of cooking, also invokes alchemy (although *The Red Book* pre-dates Jung's study of alchemy).

7 Hillman gave a shorter version of this paper at the annual meeting of the Inter-Regional Society of Jungian Analysts in Birmingham, Alabama in October 1985.

8 As Adams (1996) perceptively points out, the third meaning of whiteness does not take on a positive value in any culture (such as our own) that emphasizes masculinity and heterosexuality as normative.

References

Adams, M. V. (1996). *The Multicultural Imagination: Race, Color, and the Unconscious*. London and New York: Routledge.

Auden, W. H. (1939/1991). 'In memory of Ernst Toller'. In *Collected Poems 1907–1973*. New York: Vintage.

Brown, J. (2020). 'Whitewash'. In E. M. Sanchez (Ed.), *Merriam-Webster*. https://www.merriam-webster.com/dictionary/whitewash

Carter, C. J. (2021). 'Time for space at the table: an African American-Native American analyst-in-training's first-hand reflections. A call for the IAAP to publicly dencoune (but not erase) the White supremacist writings of C.G. Jung'. *The Journal of Analytical Psychology*, 66 (1), 70–92.

Dalal F. (1998). 'Jung: A racist'. *British Journal of Psychotherapy*, 4, 263–279.

Dohe, C. B. (2016). *Jung's Wandering Archetype: Race and Religion in Analytical Psychology*. London and New York: Routledge.

Douglas, C. (1997). 'Introduction'. In Douglas, C. (Ed.) *Visions: Notes of the Seminar Given in 1930–1934*. Princeton, NJ: Princeton University Press.

Florestal, M. (2014). *Healing Racism's Psychic Wound: A Jungian Approach*. Unpublished manuscript.

Freud, S. (1909). 'Analysis of a phobia in a five-year-old boy'. *Standard Edition 10*.

Frosh, S. (2013). *Hauntings: Psychoanalysis and Ghostly Transmissions*. London: Palgrave Macmillan.

Gerson, S. (2016). 'Afterward'. In Harris, A. and Margery Kalb, Susan Klebanoff (Eds.) *Ghosts in the Consulting Room: Echoes of Trauma in Psychoanalysis*. New York: Routledge.

Harris, A. (2012). 'The House of Difference, or White Silence'. *Studies in Gender and Sexuality*, 13, 197–216.

Hillman, J. (1986). 'Notes on White Supremacy'. *Spring: An Annual of Archetypal Psychology and Jungian Thought*.

Hillman, J. (1979). *The Dream and the Underworld*. New York: Harper Perennial.

Hillman, J. (2014). *Alchemical Psychology*. Putnum, CT: Spring Publications.

Hillman, J. & Shamdasani, S. (2013). *Lament of the Dead: Psychology after Jung's Red Book*. New York and London: W. W. Norton & Company.

Hollis, J. (2013/2015). *Hauntings: Dispelling the Ghosts Who Run Our Lives*. Asheville, NC: Chiron Publications.

Jung, C. G. (1961/2011). *Memories, Dreams, and Reflections*. New York: Vantage Books.

Jung, C. G. (1963/1989). *Mysterium Coniunctionis*. R. F. C. Hull, Trans. *CW 14*. Princeton University Press.

Jung, C. G. (1997). *Visions: Notes of the Seminar Given in 1930–1934*. C. Douglas, Ed. Princeton, NJ: Princeton University Press.

Jung, C. G. (2009). *The Red Book: A Reader's Edition*. U. Kyburz, J. Peck, and S. Shamdasani, Trans. S. Shamdasani, Ed. New York and London: W. W. Norton & Company.

Jung, C. G. (2020). *The Black Books (1913–1932): Notebooks of Transformation*. M. Liebscher, Peck, John, and Shamdasani, Sonu, Trans.; S. Shamdasani, Ed. Vol. 5. New York and London: W. W. Norton & Company.

Kearney, R. (2003). *Strangers, Gods, and Monsters: Interpreting Otherness*. New York and London: Routledge.

Kimbles, S. L. (2021). *Intergeneration Complexes in Analytical Psychology: The Suffering of Ghosts*. London and New York: Routledge.

Lamborn, A. B. (2014). 'The deus absconditus and the post-secular quest'. *Jung in the Academy and Beyond*, eds.M. F. Mattson, H. Fogarty, M. Klenck, and B. Zabriskie. New Orleans, LA: Spring Journal, Inc.

Loewald, H. W. (1980). *Papers on Psychoanalysis*. New Haven, CT: Yale University Press.

Morgan, H. (2004). 'Exploring racism'. *The Cultural Complex: Contemporary Jungian Perspectives on Psyche and Society*, eds.T. Singer & S. L. Kimbles. London and New York: Brunner-Routledge.

Morgan, H. (2021). *The Work of Whiteness: A Psychoanalytic Perspective*. London and New York: Routledge.

Obama, B. & Springsteen, B. (2021). 'Springsteen and Obama on friendship and fathers'. *The Guardian*, 23 October.

'Open letter from a group of Jungians on the question of Jung's writings on and theories about "Africans"'. (2018). *British Journal of Psychotherapy*, 34, 4, 673–678.

Plato. (1997). *Timaeus*, trans. D. Zeyl. Indianapolis, IN: Hackett Publishing Company, Inc.

Slattery, D. P. (2011). 'Thirteen ways of looking at *The Red Book*'. *Jung Journal: Culture & Psyche*, 5, 3, 128–144.

Ulanov, A. B. (2013). *Madness and Creativity*. Carolyn and Ernest Fay Series in Analytical Psychology. College Station, TX: Texas A&M University Press.

Vaughn, A. G.(2019). 'African American cultural history and reflections on Jung in the African Diaspora'. *Journal of Analytical Psychology*, 64, 3, 320–348.

Chapter 6

The Whiteness Complex
Breaking the spell

John Michael Hayes

Introduction

In writing his acclaimed *Stamped From The Beginning: The Definitive History of Racist Ideas in America,* Ibram X. Kendi concluded with these hopeful words:

> And that day is sure to come. No power lasts forever. There will come a time when Americans will realize that the only thing wrong with Black people is that they think something is wrong with Black people. There will come a time when racist ideas will no longer obstruct us from seeing the complete and utter abnormality of racial disparities. There will come a time when we will love humanity, when we will gain the courage to fight for an equitable society for our beloved humanity, knowing, intelligently, that when we fight for humanity, we are fighting for ourselves. There will come a time. Maybe, just maybe that time is now.
>
> (Kendi 2016, p. 511)

Sadly, that day has not come. Indeed, that day seems farther away than ever. Kendi's book (2016) was written before the fateful election of Donald Trump would dash any hope of authentic collective change in America.

I write this in May 2022, a week after an eighteen-year-old man went into a grocery store on a Sunday morning in Buffalo, New York and heinously shot thirteen defenseless Black people. The apprehended suspect claimed he was acting to stop colored people from replacing white people in America. This replacement theory has many adherents and is dangerously spouted in right-wing media. It represents only the most noxious and lethal exaggeration of the *"whiteness"* complex that pervades American society for most (if not all) of its existence. Contrary to Kendi's vision of a new age of racial justice and brotherhood, America is more polarized than ever.

Americans are born into a shadow history of cruelty and an exploitive abuse of power that sharply contradicts its humane, aspirational ideals enshrined in our founding documents. Our history bears witness to the genocidal elimination

DOI: 10.4324/9781003311447-7

of indigenous communities, the obscene cruelties of chattel slavery, the legacy of Jim Crow laws, segregation, and lynchings. Predatory policing, excessive and arbitrary incarceration, and systemic predatory economic and social policies have left many Black communities as blighted "sacrifice zones", districts purposefully disavowed, ignored, and abandoned to crime and decay by larger society and the political and corporate powers that be (Hedges and Sacco 2012, p. 226). Every American city has 'sacrifice zones', those communities of color that white folks blithely whizz by on their commutes to and from work in the city. These places lack decent housing, education, healthcare, even basic amenities like banks and grocery stores. The *whiteness complex* maintains an innocence of these unflattering realities and the historical and structural decisions that created them. Rather, the whiteness complex supports the comforting illusion of inherent and unmerited superiority and goodness of the white majority.

Many Americans congratulated themselves on the election of Barack Obama (4 November 2008), the first Black president, naively believing that milestone signaled an evolution into a more just, united, post-racial society. They were abruptly shocked by the virulent and aggressive reassertion of the *whiteness complex* unleashed in the Trump years (2017–2021). Perhaps that resurgence of racism was necessary, as it was lamentably predictable. Obama's election was undoubtedly an important milestone, but authentic transformation of the collective psyche demands much deeper individual and collective soul-searching, and honest confrontation with history. There can be no future peace until we Americans unflinchingly face our original sin, our grave collective shadow. Unless we find ways to break the spell of the "whiteness" complex and confront the unflattering evil of the past and present, in all its depth and complexity, there will be no justice or genuine peace. Near the end of his tragically short life, Martin Luther King, Jr. ominously and trenchantly wrote:

> If Western civilization does not now respond constructively to the challenge to banish racism, some future historian will have to say that a great civilization died because it lacked the soul and commitment to make justice a reality for all men.
>
> (King 1968, pp. 186–187)

The whiteness complex

When the French West Indian psychiatrist Frantz Fanon wrote, 'The white man is locked in his whiteness' (Fanon 1966, xiii), he named the collective complex that determines meaning and value in the white imaginary. We are born into a history that we neither chose nor *would* choose. We are thrown into unique and particular circumstances of birth, family, culture, class, language, along with our given constitution (e.g., inborn temperament and talents), and the raw psychic material of innate archetypal imperatives. Desire, action, experience and dynamics of projection and internalization create the architecture of our psyches, our personal and collective identities, and our assumptions about others's identities. Most often, we naively experience this subjectively created and constructed reality as real and factual. We live, mostly unknowingly, in the language of the self-generated, unexamined collective narratives of our tribes. Experiential life is created and dominated *by* and *in* the autonomous self-states that Carl Jung named *complexes*.

The complex is a distinctive feature and a core concept in Jungian psychology. Jung described the complex as a kind of splinter psyche: an autonomous, unreflective, unconscious self-state, marked by characteristic images, ideas, attitudes, and affects, and emerging around an archetypal core. We develop complexes around universal human existential experiences of archetypal realities, such as experiences of mother, father, siblings, power, tribe, etc.). By many decades, Jung's complex theory presciently anticipates theories of psychological multiplicity characteristic of much of contemporary relational theory that names discontinuous *self-states*—rather than internal neurotic conflict—as the basis of psychological organization.

Importantly, Jung writes: 'What is not so well known, though far more important theoretically, is that complexes can *have us*. The existence of complexes throws serious doubt on the naïve assumption of the unity of consciousness, which is equated with the "psyche" and on the supremacy of the will' (Jung 1948, p.96). Jung also writes: "The *via regia* to the unconscious … is not the dream … but the complex, which is the architect of dreams and symptoms. Nor is this *via* very royal' (ibid., p.101), and, 'Where the realm of the complexes begins, the freedom of the ego comes to an end' (ibid., p.104).

When in the grip of a complex, we unknowingly experience selected aspects of internal and external reality and disavow other aspects. To be in the grip of a complex is to be under a spell. The complex not only determines experience of current reality, but also affects the cast of our memories of past events and relationships. This is an important key to understanding the way in which the 'whiteness' complex alters people's understanding of history in some sectors, in flagrant disregard for established fact, to maintain the preferred myth of white superiority and specialness. Witness the feverish revolt against the prospect of teaching Critical Race Theory in some districts, and the fear that children and adolescents will no longer be inducted into the comforting myths of "whiteness".

Complexes are the natural way that we organize and experience psychological life. Complexes can be positive or negative; they are only problematic when they have a rigid hold on the psyche and when we are unable to break the spell of the complex, to recognize with self-awareness that the the complex is just a complex, and to thereby open up degrees of psychological freedom, meaning, and awareness. Complexes are most rigidly held and deeply entrenched when there is trauma or threat. Many experience the growing changes in the ethnic composition of the nation as a mortal threat to the myth of "whiteness". For this reason, the celebrated Obama victory was experienced as an existential defeat by those deep in the grip of the "whiteness" complex.

A complex effectively creates a particular experiential reality, and blocks out and disavows contradictory and challenging realities. Ta-Nahesi Coates describes the 'white imaginary' as that habitual state of mind and feeling of self-satisfaction and unchallenged superiority in white people, that disavows those inconvenient, horrifically unflattering facts of American history that challenge and disturb this image:

> But race is the child of racism, not the father. And the process of naming "the people" has never been a matter of genealogy and physiognomy so much as one of hierarchy. Difference in hue and hair is old. But the belief in the pre-eminence of hue and hair, and the notion that these factors can correctly organize a society and that they signify deeper attributes, which are indelible—this is the new idea at the heart of these new people who have been brought up hopelessly, tragically, deceitfully, to believe that they are white.
>
> (Coates 2015, p. 7)

When Ta Nehisi Coates names the "white imaginary", that semi-hypnotic state of mind that disavows discomforting history of violent and exploitive oppression and indulges unexamined fantasies of white supremacy and superiority, he is alluding to that which I identify as the *whiteness complex*.

Author, educator, and public speaker Jennifer Harvey described an exercise with groups of Black and white church people in *Dear White Christians* (2014). The Black people were asked to name the things about being "Black" that made them proud. Without hesitation, they listed a dozen positive qualities: resilience, perseverance, warmth, humor, etc. In contrast, the white folks were disorganized and flummoxed when asked to name positive qualities of being "white". Some in this group responded by naming qualities of their Jewish, Irish, and Italian ethnicities ... they substituted a more comfortable question for the difficult one. The request to name positive things about being white met with a prolonged, embarrassed, and awkward silence. The question evoked profound anxiety and emotional dissociation (Harvey 2014, p. 63).

Harvey's experience mirrors Jung's research with the Word Association Test in which he identified and defined the *complex* phenomenon. Patients were asked to respond to a stimulus word (e.g., dog, house, streetcar, mother, etc.) with the first word that came to mind. More telling than the content of the response was the time delay in answering. Significant response latency indicated that the stimulus word touched a conflicted, troublesome, underlying complex. Jung understood the complex as a network of thoughts, feelings, affects, memories connected by associative links. Jung understood personality as a loose network of complexes, each with distinctive physiological and psychological signature, and each creating a distinct experiential reality in the individual. The more the complex was complicated by trauma, painful conflict, and disturbing affect, the more the complex came to be dissociated, having an autonomous existence as a splinter psyche. To be "in a complex" is to have one's emotional and mental reality shaped by that complex. The complex's spell is particularly strong when associated with painful, disturbing images, thoughts, and feelings. Harvey's meeting with silence and dissociation suggests something about the depth, complexity, and the fragility of the *whiteness complex.*

Educator Robin Di Angelo writes that this white fragility in confronting racial differences stems from unexamined, unearned privilege:

> Socialized into a deeply internalized sense of superiority that we either are unaware of or can never admit to ourselves, we become highly fragile in conversations about race. We consider a challenge to our racial worldviews as a challenge to our very identities as good, moral people.
>
> (DiAngelo 2018, p. 1)

Identifying the concept of the complex neither keeps one from having a complex nor does it prevent one from being under the cultural complex's spell. Indeed, Jung's writings are riddled with repetitive, casual, Eurocentric assumptions of the moral, cognitive, and psychological superiority of his own "race" (Dalal 1988; Carter 2021). This is evident in his condescending reference to 'negroes', and other so-called 'primitives'. Jung is hardly distinct in being under the spell of a Eurocentric, colonialist mentality—a cultural complex of *whiteness*—in his perceptions and assumptions about peoples whom he neither really knew nor understood. One cannot know the other unless the complex is recognized for its limitations and is then transcended. In this, Jung was not only regrettably "all-too-human" and a "man-of-his-time". Not all his contemporaries shared his blindness in this area. It has been said that great men have great shadows. Despite some glaring lacunae, Jung was prescient in identifying the spiritual bankruptcy of the West and he was prophetic in acknowledging our urgent need for an awakened consciousness. Whatever his personal failings and limitations, Jung accurately diagnosed the spiritual malady of western culture and its impending consequences.

In America, a viable future can only be had when the hold of the *whiteness complex* is broken. There can be no future justice and peace in a country that will not own up to its shadow, its past and present racial evils. Jung's theory gives us conceptual tools to understand our predicament and hopefully to find a way forward.

This chapter attempts to use Jungian concepts of the complex (as it lives within the individual and within the collective) to analyze and deconstruct America's systemic racism. Systemic racism is hardly an exclusively American problem. Recent history makes clear America is still very much entrenched in its particularly vicious brand of racism. The roots of racism go deep and wide, infecting every aspect of American culture. Reasonably aware and benevolent people easily dis-identify with the resurgent crude racism that is on common display. There are deeper levels of unrecognized and unacknowledged, subtle and more insidious racism that infects all aspects of American life, including religious communities, universities, and psychoanalytic institutes. The urgent self-scrutiny this demands has begun in many of these institutions. The whiteness complex's poisonous spell must be broken if our nation can thrive and fulfill any of its promise.

The *cultural complex*

Jung's concept of the complex has been extended from individual psychology toward understanding group psychology and culture. The whiteness complex has a hold on individuals as individuals; but it is also a 'cultural complex' that has a noxious hold on the group mind of culture (Henderson 1984; Adams 1996). Jungian analyst Helen Morgan usefully observed that psychoanalytic perspectives on racism apply the concepts of projection, splitting, and introjection, concepts developed in the study of individual psychopathology. While these are somewhat useful, they do not capture the cultural dimension of racism, i.e., the manner in which *whiteness* shapes and limits awareness and how it is enacted reflexively and behaviorally in collective customs and habits of thought, language, and action (Morgan 2021, p. 88).

Philosopher Linda Alcoff (2015) described the deep and pervasive embeddedness of the complex: '"Whiteness" is lived and not merely represented. It is a prominent feature of one's way of being in the world, of how one navigates that world and of how one is navigated around by others' (Alcoff 2015, p. 9). Alcoff observed that whites resist this formulation, being unaccustomed—as minority groups are not—to the implied limitation on individual choice in this description of their group mind (ibid., p. 21). Alcoff also alludes to the epistemic set of the *whiteness complex's* assertion that society is essentially a fair meritocracy, Black people are the reason for their own troubles, and racism is a thing of the past (ibid., p. 84).

In their introduction to *The Cultural Complex* (2004), Thomas Singer and Samuel L. Kimbles make the critical point that having a cultural complex is an unavoidable part of being human. Cultural and individual complexes are problematic when they are the sole basis of identity: 'there is a healthy cultural identity (or 'cultural ego') that can clearly be seen as separate from the more negative and contaminating aspects of cultural complexes' (p.5). Awareness of the complex on an individual or collective basis and understanding its determinants and its influence breaks the spell of the complex and opens up degrees of freedom for broader consciousness and relationality.

Archetypes of the whiteness complex: blackness, hierarchy, and the scapegoat

The seed of the complex is the *archetype*, a Jungian concept sometimes misunderstood as an inherited idea or image. An archetype is the innate human potential to form typical, affectively charged images in universal life-stages. Jung writes about the relation of an archetype to experience as a complex develops:

> The form of the world into which he is born is already inborn in him as virtual image. Likewise parents, wife, children, birth, and death are inborn in him as virtual images, as psychic aptitudes. These *a priori* categories have by nature a collective character; they are images of parents, wife, and children in general and are not individual predestinations. We must therefore think of these images as lacking in solid content, hence as unconscious. They only acquire solidity, influence, and eventual conscious-ness in the encounter with empirical facts, which touch the unconscious aptitude and quicken it to life.

> (Jung 1938, para. 300)

As the name implies, a complex is a multi-dimensional, multiply determined cluster of images, attitudes, and affects that emerges and evolves around archetypal ideas and images sparked in fateful moments of encounter with existential realities (Shalit 2002). We know that whiteness and blackness are socially and culturally constructed phenomena, having no empirical basis in biological differences. I identify three related archetypal images that are implicit in the whiteness complex: blackness, hierarchy, and scapegoating.

As a white person trying to shed the remnants of the whiteness complex's hold, I reflect on early life experiences that quickened my unconscious potential to experience *blackness*, hierarchy and scapegoating, and brought them to life in my psyche. These formed my initiation into the whiteness complex.

When I was a young boy, my entire extended family lived in the Bedford-Stuyvesant section of Brooklyn. My parents were the grandchildren of immigrants who fled the horror and decimation of nineteenth-century Ireland. My great grandparents, grandparents, aunts, and uncles all made their home in our neighborhood. In the 1950s, the neighborhood was rapidly becoming a destination for new exiles—Black folks fleeing the Jim Crow south, part of the great migration northward that Isabelle Wilkerson describes in *The Warmth of Other Suns* (2010).

A bright, sensitive boy of seven, I was hardly aware of the history I in-habited. I had only hints of harsh realities beneath the cordial surfaces of our shared urban village. I certainly recognized that some friends had darker skin and curly hair, but I was only vaguely aware this carried any significance.

Certainly, there were implicitly racist structures that made deep impressions. Black and white folks lived next door to each other, did not live in the same buildings. Within fifty feet of each other, there were two "separate but equal" Catholic churches, each with their own rectory, convent, and parochial school. As children, we negotiated all these spaces together, playing in each other's homes, backyards, and schools. Nevertheless, I was stunned to learn my *whiteness* and their *blackness* had terribly significant implications I did not yet recognize or understand.

My friend Danny, who was Black, and I went to the candy store at the end of our block to spend our nickels. We were not there for very long when the storeowner angrily and abruptly accused Danny of stealing candy. The storeowner made Danny empty his pockets there and then to prove his protested innocence. Danny's pockets were empty. No apologies were offered. I felt a hot flush of anger and shame, and shame at my own stunned powerlessness. Danny seemed nonplussed, as if he had been through this before and almost expected such suspicion. It then dawned on me that I had a privilege of presumed innocence that Danny would never share. My *whiteness* was a privilege that I guiltily embraced even as I was impotently furious at the injustice of Danny's disadvantage. Complicated feelings took hold. I felt shame for the enjoyment of my unearned superior status. I felt both guilt and relief that I was spared Danny's fate. This might have been the formative moment when it dawned on me that I inherited a superior place in the collective hierarchy, as *blackness* inexplicably carried a negative stigma.

Hierarchy is an inescapable archetypal dimension of group life and culture with which I was well acquainted. A skinny and awkward boy, I knew the shame of being picked last in pick-up games of stickball. Hierarchical status was supposed to be conferred by one's demonstrated ability (or lack thereof). Instinctively, I knew that there was something sinister about an unmerited hierarchy that is based on race, embraced and enjoyed without deliberate consideration.

Concepts of hierarchy are archetypally driven ideas that structure human groups. Ideas of who is "up" and who is "down"—who is superior and who is inferior—are universal mental structures created by lived experience in the culture we inhabit. In *Race: A Theological Account* (2008), J. Kameron Carter discusses how Gnosticism, in both its ancient and modern forms, creates assumptions of a clear hierarchy of the value for human beings. Jung adopted many Gnostic assumptions into his psychology. Perhaps Jung did not realize that he had unexamined prejudices, not seeing beyond his own cultural complex. James Baldwin trenchantly illuminated America's unconscious hierarchy:

> There are too many things that we do not wish to know about ourselves. People are not … terribly anxious to be equal (equal, after all, to what and to whom?) but they love the idea of being superior. And this human truth

has an especially grinding force here, where people are perpetually attempting to find their feet on the shifting sands of status.

(Baldwin 1963, p. 88)

There is no conception of black without a conception of white. But these terms have acquired racial meanings and mental associations in western culture. As a black West Indian psychiatrist living in France, Franz Fanon wrote about the pathology of the white imagination of the Black man as dangerous, aggressive, with a dark, superior phallic prowess that evokes fear, fascination and envy in whites:

In Europe, evil is symbolized by the black man ... the perpetrator is the black man: Satan is black; one talks of darkness; when your are filthy you are dirty—and this goes for physical dirt as well as moral dirt ... In Europe, the black man, whether physically or symbolically, represents the dark side of the personality ... Darkness, obscurity, shadow, gloom, night, the labyrinth of the underworld, the murky depths, blackening someone's reputation ... the black man symbolizes sin. The archetype of inferior values is represented by the black man.

(Fanon 1966, p. 165)

Fanon agrees with Jung that this accurately describes an archetype in the white psychological imaginary. But Fanon criticizes Jung's "big mistake" in universalizing and concretizing this collective complex. *Blackness* does not carry the negative, shadow qualities for all peoples outside of the western world (Fanon 1966, p. 166).

Jung emphasizes that all archetypes are bipolar, having two poles of meaningful associational networks. The negative associations to *blackness* are countered by positive images of depth, of mystery, of warmth, etc. Positive associations to *whiteness* in the western imaginary include images of *innocence, purity, light*, etc. Jungian analyst James Hillman (1986) emphasized that there is also a negative pole of associations to white: blankness, pallid color, death, cowardice, etc. But few have the ability to stand in the tension of opposites and comprehend the whole reality, but that is necessary to transcend the complex. Breaking the spell of the *whiteness complex* necessitates outgrowing the immature tendency to experience and identify with only one of the split polarities. In his last major work Jung wrote:

The tendency to separate the opposites as much as possible and to strive for singleness of meaning is absolutely necessary for clarity of consciousness, since discrimination is of its essence. But when the separation is carried so far that the complementary opposite is lost sight of, and the blackness of the whiteness, the evil of the good, the depth of the heights, and so on, is no longer seen, the result is one-sidedness, which is then compensated from the unconscious without our help. The counterbalancing is even done against our will, which in consequence must become more and more fanatical until it brings about a catastrophic enantiodroma. Wisdom never forgets that all things have two sides, and it would also know how to avoid such calamities if ever it had any power. But power is never found in the seat of wisdom; it is always the focus of mass interest and is therefore inevitably associated with the illimitable folly of the mass man.

(Jung 1963, pp. 333–34)

Race is a socially constructed reality, invented to serve and justify nefarious ends. To describe people as *white* and *black* is a false dichotomy, a duplicitous opposition of opposites. These so-called opposites of white and black do not exist in a tension that needs to be born, so much as that tension needs to be collapsed and discarded. There are no *white* or *black* people. Human beings come in all the various and varying shades of brown. There is one race, the Human Race.

The scapegoating pattern in the whiteness complex is also sadly archetypal. Rene Girard (1978) regards the scapegoat dynamic as the key to understanding human collective behavior. Girard's theory is complex and profound in its implications and can only be alluded to here. While Girard makes no allusion to Jung in his writings, the scapegoating dynamic he describes is clearly archetypal. Girard describes a pattern of mimetic desire and rivalry that threatens group cohesion and safety with violence. The identification of a scapegoat provides a kind of safety valve for the group tension that threatens to break into violence. The excited camaraderie in identifying the scapegoat and making that person or group the target of group violence is infectious and numinous. The violent enactment becomes memorialized in myth and religion. This archetypal scapegoating dynamic underlies the worst chapters of all human history. American history is no exception.

A few years of childhood feels like a long time. My young life was caught up in the nexus of two large post-war American social movements in New York City: the Black migration north and the migration of white folks out of the old ethnic neighborhoods to Long Island. Our new home in Rosedale at the far southeastern corner of Queens was made up almost exclusively of Jewish, Italian, and Irish ex-pat Brooklynites. There were no Black people in Rosedale. It was not something that was thought about or discussed. No one thought anything of this. Their evident absence was collectively disavowed. Black people were left behind in Brooklyn. Implicitly, it was recognized that this distance was supposed to be an improvement.

It is noteworthy that post-war American Jews, Italians, and Irish people were relatively recently granted the status of being unambiguously included in the category of "white". Each of these ethnic groups had their own particular narratives of trauma, dispossession, and devaluation inflicted by those higher up in the social hierarchy. That history rarely impelled empathy for the struggle of Black people for inclusion and dignity. Signs that read "No dogs, no jews, no irish, no blacks" were not rare at places of employment and housing in New York well into the early twentieth century. Reactively and defensively, these groups jealously guarded their *whiteness* (their differences from Blacks) and were all too happy to have a ready scapegoat to reinforce their shaky senses of social identity and status.

Decades after leaving home, I was a graduate student living in Philadelphia. One evening, I was stunned to happen upon Bill Moyers's hour-long documentary (1976) that exposed how Rosedale's implicit racism broke out into violent conflict. Those few and intrepid Black families who initially bought homes in Rosedale were welcomed with firebombing and death threats. Hierarchy, when threatened, quickly morphs into scapegoating violence. Here were the folks I grew up among, spewing vicious and violent hatred of Black newcomers. Their unapologetic and feverish attack on these new neighbors spawned a renewed sense of intense community and camaraderie, just as Girard described. It is quite disturbing but hardly surprising that *white* children joined in the violent scapegoating of *Black* children. One Black child interviewed remarked,

They treat us like we're a piece of dirt, dogs ... I mean that's the way you treat an animal. I mean, God, we're human beings. You don't treat other people like that, it's just wrong. Black, white I don't care. A person is a person. Skin should have no bearing on how you treat a person. That's just wrong.

(Moyers 1976)

Breaking the spell of whiteness

Breaking the whiteness complex will require much more than liberal good intentions and interracial fellowship. As Kendi asserted, racism is not going to disappear merely by white people getting greater exposure to relationships with Black people. It is also clear that racism is not going to be dispelled merely by educational means. Those well-intentioned liberal attempts not only do not work, but also inadvertently serve the purposes of maintaining the *whiteness complex*. The whiteness complex is not a relational problem to be resolved with Black people; it is a serious white problem. It is a most dangerous limitation of white people in America. This white problem demands internal reckoning with America's shameful history of structurally exploitive injustice to Black people, and our individual and collective privileges. Nothing less than deep, sustained, unflinching, and authentic reckoning can begin to dislodge the hold of the whiteness complex.

In the late 1970s, I moved to Columbia, Maryland, a progressive new community between Washington, D.C. and Baltimore. Columbia was deliberately designed to counter racial and economic segregation. Here, I have lived and have raised my family. This social experiment had some relative success. I was pleased to have Black neighbors and for my children to have friends of both *races*. But when I reflect on those years, I wonder how much of the good feelings were those of a kind of *noblesse oblige* that left the assumption of white superiority unexamined and unchallenged. We could congratulate ourselves for being socially progressive and inclusive, but from a place of generous superiority that kept the whiteness complex intact. Columbia was a liberal version of Coates's "white imaginary", which he describes as that state of mind that disavows history, privilege, and responsibility, and maintains a safe distance from the terrible problems of the inner city that were largely created and maintained by white oppression and exploitation. The blighted neighborhoods of Coates's boyhood home in West Baltimore are a scant fifteen miles from the leafy vales of Columbia, and yet a world away.

If the whiteness complex has deeper unconscious roots that will not be touched by relational experience or educational means, neither will it be dispelled by politics. Kendi maintains that an America free of racism must involve both a radical change of consciousness and a shift in power:

> Power will never self-sacrifice away from its self-interest. Power cannot be persuaded away from its self-interest. Power cannot be educated away from its self-interest. … An antiracist America can only be guaranteed if principled antiracists are in power, and then antiracist policies become the law of the land and then antiracist ideas become the common sense of the people, and then the antiracist common sense of the people holds those antiracist leaders and policies accountable.'
>
> (Kendi 2016, pp. 508–10)

That is true as far as it goes; but shifts in political power will not result in the deep change in consciousness that is necessary for real transformation. A political shift in power does not necessarily change consciousness. Eight years of the Obama presidency—a presidency characterized by exemplary rectitude and competence—exacerbated rather than dispelled the hold of the *whiteness complex* in many people. Any Trump rally or alt-right gathering demonstrates that the group camaraderie and identity in triumph that are the marks of scapegoating violence against Black people are again sadly all too evident in American life.

Girard maintains that the only way to break out of the hold of that scapegoating mechanism is by deepening empathy for the victims of violence. Although feeling for the other is a mark of empathy, essentially empathy is an act of perception and cognition: to perceive and know the other's experience from their perspective, to identify with the plight of the scapegoated victim.

This necessarily involves a decentering of oneself from one's mythic assumptions and recognizing them for what they are. It assumes the psychological maturity to 'mentalize' one's own thoughts and feelings, i.e., to recognize one's internal narratives as subjectively created and maintained narratives, and to simultaneously recognize the validity of the subjectively created reality of the other (Fonagy et al. 2002). That maturity is not abundantly in evidence. The capacity to maintain a mind of one's own is always a fragile developmental achievement. We humans are all too vulnerable to regress to mob mentality and scapegoating violence.

To be valid and productive, white empathy for the experience of Black people cannot and must not attempt to thereby evade responsibility and acknowledgement of the horrific realities of history, past and present. That history is always "in the room" in white encounters with Black people, whether or not that is inconvenient.

My first experience as a new and late-ordained Episcopal priest was to assist at a church in West Baltimore that was attempting to become a genuinely interracial community dedicated to the glaring needs of the surrounding area. Black and white folks from very different backgrounds managed to get to know each other and work together. No one had any illusions that building trust would be easily achieved. After seven years of weekly Eucharist, countless coffee hours, meetings, picnics, baby showers, a few weddings, and funerals, it felt that some measure of community and good feeling was secured. Then abruptly, the yearly celebration of the church's namesake erupted into angry accusations and schism. The dynamics and details are more complex than can be related here. Essentially the Black folks accused the white folks of a kind of 'toxic charity' that made them feel patronized and belittled (Lupton 2012). The white folks were blindsided and angry. Both groups felt betrayed and injured. Most of the congregation drifted away over the next few months. It is beyond sad that this seemingly viable interracial church community was so fragile.

One of the major faults was that the white folks wanted to skip over the necessary step of difficult reckoning with their complicity with the history of oppression and exploitation of Black people and move seamlessly to reconciliation. The Black folks rightly perceived that white people were, in essence, using them to assuage guilt and reinforce subtly a sense of superiority. Human motivations are always complicated; but, to some extent, the otherwise well-intentioned white folks were attempting to expiate collective guilt while maintaining a stance of inherent superiority. The Black folks saw through these naïve and self-congratulatory gestures.

Breaking the spell of the "whiteness" complex is no easy matter. Nothing less than full recognition of the "whiteness" complex as a self-state, as a self-narrative, a story white folks tell ourselves to stave off facing the horrific realities of our history, can open the possibilities of authentic empathy and understanding. That will necessarily involve suffering prolonged shame, grief, and sorrow. This must be suffered. There can be no rush to forgiveness or reconciliation. Human beings have limited capacity to tolerate painful truth and the temptation to regression to tribal thinking is always present. It is not at all assured that genuine change can be achieved. A genuine breaking of the spell is not to be just a shift in internal consciousness or in-group mentality. To be real, breaking the spell must include some impetus toward reparation in whatever appropriate forms that might take.

References

Adams, M. V. (1996). *The Multicultural Imagination: "Race", Color and the Unconscious*. London & New York: Routledge Press.

Alcoff, L. M. (2015). *The Future of Whiteness*. Cambridge: Polity Press.

Baldwin, J. (1963). *The Fire Next Time*. New York: Random House.

Carter, C. J. (2021). 'Time for Space at the Table: An African American-Native American Analyst-in-Training's First-Hand Reflections, A Call for the IAAP to Publicly Denounce (But Not Erase) the White Supremacist Writings of C. G. Jung'. *Journal of Analytical Psychology* 66:70–92.

Carter, J. K. (2008). *Race: A Theological Account*. Oxford & New York: Oxford University Press.

Coates, T. (2015). *Between The World And Me*. New York: One World.

Dalal, F. (1988). 'Jung: A Racist'. *British Journal of Psychotherapy* 4(3): 263–279.

DiAngelo, R. (2018). *White Fragility: Why It's So Hard to Talk About Racism*. Boston: Beacon Press.

Fanon, F. (1952). *Black Skin, White Masks*. R. Philcox, trans. New York: Grove Press.

Fonagy, P., Gyorgy, G., Jurist, E. & Target, M. (2002). *Affect Regulation, Mentalization, and the Development of Self*. New York: Other Press.

Girard, R. (1978). *Things Hidden Since the Foundation of the World*. S. Bann and M. Metteer, trans. Stanford: Stanford University Press.

Harvey, J. (2014). *Dear White Christians: For Those Still Longing for Racial Reconciliation*. Grand Rapids: Wm. Eerdmans Publishing.

Hedges, C. & Sacco, J. (2012). *Days of Destruction Days of Revolt*. New York: Nations Press.

Henderson, J. (1984). *Cultural Attitudes in Psychological Perspective*. New York: Inner City Press.

Hillman, J. (1986). 'Notes on White Supremacy, Essaying an Archetypal Account of Historical Events'. Dallas: Spring Publications.

Jung, C. G. (1938). 'The Relations between the Ego and the Unconscious'. *Collected Works 7*.

Jung, C. G. (1963) 'Rex and Regina'. *CW 14*.

Jung, C. G. (1948) 'A Review of the Complex Theory'. *CW 8*.

Kendi, I. X. (2016). *Stamped from the Beginning: The Definitive History of Racist Ideas in America*. New York: Nation Books.

King, M. L., Jr. (1968). *Where Do We Go From Here: Chaos or Community?* Boston: Beacon Press.

Lupton, R. D. (2012). *Toxic Charity: How Churches and Charities Hurt Those They Help*. New York: HarperCollins Publishing.

Morgan, H. (2021). *The Work of Whiteness: A Psychological Perspective*. City: Routledge.

Moyers, B. (1976). *Rosedale: The Way It Is. Bill Moyers' Journal*.

Shalit, E. (2002). *The Complex: Path of Transformation from Archetype to Ego*. New York: Inner City Books.

Singer, T. & Kimbles, S. L. (2004). *The Cultural Complex*. New York: Brunner-Routledge.

Wilkerson, I. (2010). *The Warmth of Other Suns*. New York: Random House.

Chapter 7

The Sunken Place
Silence as the propagation of toxic whiteness

Tiffany Houck

An Eruption of Innocence

It was a beautiful summer morning. A lifelong dear friend, my daughter, and I were enjoying bagels and lox on a blanket in the park, punctuated by impromptu turns with a jump rope and a frisbee. The purpose of our breakfast picnic was to strategize a movement to build a community garden in an abandoned lot next to our building in upper Manhattan. The lot had been left untended for over twenty years. My daughter got this idea after reading a novel where a family of kids in Harlem covertly overtook an abandoned lot and created a beautiful public garden, renegade-style. This lifelong friend of mine had a prominent position in city government and had already helped my daughter build a website where people could sign a petition to support and to advocate for this garden's-creation. This friend, a Black/Puerto Rican man who was born and raised in Washington Heights (Manhattan) in the 1980s, has dedicated his life to organizing and dismantling systemic racism. The conversations the three of us shared that morning went beyond discussions of creating a public garden. The conversation sprawled into systemic issues that act as barricades against efforts to beautify poorer neighborhoods. My friend was empowering my white daughter to advocate for the construction of a public space that could act as a unifier and safe haven for the diverse populations of our neighborhood that were so effected by the Coronavirus pandemic and the uprising after the murder of George Floyd (25 May 2020). My friend was educating her about the underlying assumptions she may be bringing to the table. He was teaching her about being responsible to herself and to her ideas amidst historical and systemic racism, deep issues she was inheriting. It was such a rich morning of learning, planning, and being together. At one point, we had a gaggle of children taking turns jumping Double-Dutch as my friend and I continued our conversation. My daughter followed her eleven-year-old impulse to run-off and play with others as my friend and I spoke about the complications of working toward more just and equitable ways of living.

DOI: 10.4324/9781003311447-8

The Sunken Place 115

After a long, luxurious morning of playing and planning, the three of us gathered up our belongings and headed for home. On the way out of the park, I noticed a handful of Latinx children digging around this big tree. These were the same children who had joined us for Double-Dutch just moments beforehand. They looked as if they were preparing to plant something. I off-handedly commented to my daughter, 'You should hire them to help you with your garden!' My friend stopped in his tracks and stopped me in mine. 'There it is, right there,' he said to me. It took me a minute to even realize to what he was referring. 'White supremacy, in action'. Instead of seeing these children as collaborators, fellow organizers, neighbors, I saw them as "hired help". I was shocked by my unconscious and automatic comment. I was even more shocked by my ignorance, having been blind to the implications of what I had said until my friend called me out. As Helen Morgan says,

> White privilege does not require people's conscious awareness for it to exist; indeed, its very invisibility is key to its continuance as it allows us the freedom to be blind to our own privilege … . Our inability (or refusal) to see how privileged our position is allows us not only to enjoy our racial advantages but to persist in defending them.
>
> (Morgan 2021, p. 17)

I lead with this vignette to touch within myself that which is so slippery in the topic at hand. The very thing I seek to address—*toxic whiteness* and its effects on the analytic project—is written from a position of power and privilege. I want to name this before I begin. There are dynamics at the archetypal core of white supremacy that I wish to amplify. These are dynamics that are not unfamiliar to me. I feel neither immune nor somehow above these dynamics. This is my starting place.

Get Out: An Amplification on the Horror of Dissociation in the White Imaginary

Aside from his friend's warning and his own dawning awareness that things are not as they seem, Chris, the protagonist in the movie *Get Out* (2017) pleads with his believed-to-be girlfriend (Rose, the antagonist) for the keys to the car … his one hope for escape from the house of horror. He seeks the keys to his libidinal vehicle of liberation. At the climax of Jordan Peele's film, *Get Out*, Chris simultaneously realizes that the entire weekend at his (white) girlfriend's parent's house and his relationship to Rose are all a set-up to trap him and to sell his body to the highest white bidder. It is modern-day slave trade in which the subject is paraded about shackled to the unknown chains of psychic possession in lieu of the auctioneer's block.

This poignant film was released one year after Trump's election ignited a surge of overtly racialized hate crimes across America. In response to overt racialization, the Black Lives Matter movement strengthened during this period. We witness something more horrifying than traditional horror—nice, white, Obama-voting liberals have devised a new plantation. Black bodies are revered, sought after, desired, and seemingly protected, all for the sake of the white psyche, the perpetuation of whiteness within the black body. The black body is revered and elevated and then insidiously occupied by white desire. The black body is objectified as strong, sexual, capable, sought after for longevity, youth, and beauty. It is to be colonized and occupied by aging and ailing white bodies who seek a fantasied fountain of youth.

Peele depicts a new form of slave-trade ritual that takes place at the house of the Kincaide family, where annual modern "slave auction" parties are hosted. Before the weekend's slave trade begins, Rose's mother, Missy (a psychiatrist) induces a conditioned automatic state of paralysis in Chris (the protagonist). With a tap on her teacup, she thrusts Chris into *the sunken place*, a place of immobile liminality, of falling forever. Chris is suspended in nothingness, screaming with no one to hear him. Meanwhile, the watching audience peer down upon him. Missy will later hand him over to her husband. A neurosurgeon, her husband will remove a portion of Chris's brain (keeping his body alive) to replace it with the cognitive functioning and memory network system of the brain of the highest white bidder seeking the fountain of youth. The previously white-bodied individual is to be endowed with a longer life in a stronger body. The white person's brain will occupy the black body, leaving only a small trace of his own psyche behind the eyes of his new inhabitant.

Throughout the film, we receive glimpses of the former psyche of the Black subject whose body was abducted and sold, when, certain brief flickers of light cause a glitch in the system. The Black psyche is contacted and momentarily erupts in outrageous fear and tries to escape. It desperately urges Chris to GET OUT, only to be thrust back into paralysis by the psychiatrist mother. One can feel the truth of these scenes cloaked within this horror film.

Peele readily employs horror to amplify an experience of being Black in a world of good white liberals. Simultaneously, Peele draws out the unconscious enactment of silence and paralysis that is often the result of the white imaginary. Claudia Rankine introduced the concept of the racial imaginary as a biproduct of culturally constructed biases that live within the imagination and inform the very desire of the one who wishes to write about or create works of art pertaining to "race". Her inquiries led to her book *The Racial Imaginary* (2015), written in conjunction with Beth Loffreda. I suggest Rankine's concept of the racial imaginary helps us understand the operation at the Kincaide compound. In their imagining the Black subject, they can objectify the black body and distance themselves from their own implication in the most horrific acts.

In Peele's film, we watch white people hungrily, silently bidding over the young and strong black body—not to relate to it but to colonize it, use it, and own it from the inside-out based on their own imaging of its bounty. The instrument that the psychiatrist (Missy) uses thrusts her Black subject into this place of utter suspension and near annihilation. I suggest that Peele's *sunken place* might be understood as his portrayal of one of the effects that the white imaginary has upon the Black experience. The tool used by the white psychiatrist (Missy) to help "address his childhood trauma" and to help rid Chris of his smoking habit is a tool of the white imaginary. The white subject believes that she knows better and then uses that knowing to rob the subject of his own volition, threatening to lock the Black subject into a state of liminality and dissociation. I suggest that Missy's violation of Chris's volition—thrusting him into the *sunken place*—has a dual meaning. This state of paralysis in the sunken place is not only an amplification of the unconscious repetition of the effects of white silence upon the Black subject but is simultaneously an amplification of the effects of white silence upon the white subject. She thrusts Chris into the sunken place, suspended in liminality, so that she cannot hear his protest. She refuses to be affected by his subjectivity. In doing this, she evacuates her own sense of volition and claims innocence in this action. In a form of reversal, Peele portrays the violence of white silence upon the Black subject while simultaneously amplifying the violence that white silence has upon all subjects. The horror enacted on the Black subject is the result of the white subject's refusal to be penetrated by the protest of the Black subject, her silencing the reality of the other in front of her, her refusal to be implicated in her acts of violence.

Peele's film, along with the emerging cinematic genre of Black Horror (*Love Craft Country, Watchmen, Us,* and *Them* as other recent poignant examples), brings the true-to-life horror of the modern Black experience into *feeling* through the act of storytelling and mythology. In *Get Out,* the silencing of the Black subject robs him of his volition, his voice, his subjectivity; therefore, the white subject is allowed to continue acts of violence without feeling implicated. So, she simultaneously silences and shuts-off her own capacity for increased consciousness. One could argue this amplification is more relatable to the overt and conscious acts of white supremacy in our country today. This violent act of silencing the *other* into paralysis (which Peele so aptly portrays) is at play within our own field of psychoanalysis. It shows up in the guise of *analytic neutrality.* The fact that Peele uses the image of a psychiatrist as the perpetrator speaks to the dangerous reality that lives deeply within our own field of work and study—the danger of claiming psychoanalytic innocence (Sheehi & Sheehi 2021) or neutrality.

What is brilliant about Peele's rendition here is that he speaks from within the Black experience to critique an unconscious enactment of *white body supremacy* (Menakem 2017). Thrusting Black consciousness into the sunken place, seeking to eliminate it from our educational institutions, banning books by Black authors from our public libraries, and, even within institutions of psychoanalysis (Moss 2020; Zeavin 2022) are all enactments of white body supremacy in our current epoch. These enactments paralyze the processes of becoming conscious within the psyches of whites. By undermining, disregarding, and rendering impotent the Black experience as articulated by Black authors and within the concepts of Critical Race Theory itself (Iati 2021), white consciousness remains, itself, paralyzed, stunted, delayed and therefore, dangerous. The irony of Peele's image of the sunken place is that the white psychiatrist is enacting her own dissociation through the ways in which she seeks to cut off and thrust into unconsciousness that which she cannot and refuses to confront within herself. By contorting and asserting her power as the "clinical expert" over the Black subject, she asserts her power and escapes being penetrated by his truthful gaze (a photographer, Chris sees from behind the poignant lens).

The Archetypal Core of White Body Supremacy Trauma

What Peele amplifies mythologically is the psychic defense against integration within the white-bodied person that comes as a result of *white body supremacy trauma* (Menakem 2017). A clinical social worker and trauma therapist, Menakem describes *white body supremacy trauma* as unhealed racialized trauma that cannot be traced back to a single, specific event. In white bodies, it is trauma resultant from inflicting and perpetuating white supremacy in our cultural institutions and collective life in general. Charles W. Mills describes white supremacy as 'the unnamed political system that has made the modern world what it is today' (Mills 1997, p. 122). While white supremacy has shaped Western political and social thought and practices for hundreds of years, it has never been named as such. Its silence renders white supremacy unconscious and invisible unto its perpetrators. Mills argues that white supremacy's power is drawn from its very silence. Robin DiAngelo (2018) reminds us:

> race scholars use the term white supremacy to describe a sociopolitical economic system of domination based on racial categories that benefit those defined and perceived as white. This system of structural power privileges, centralizes, and elevates white people as a group.
>
> (DiAngelo 2018, p. 29)

DiAngelo uses Charles Mills to explain

> two points that are critical to our understanding of white fragility. First, white supremacy is never acknowledged. Second, we cannot study any sociopolitical system without addressing how that system is mediated by race. The failure to acknowledge white supremacy protects it from examination and holds it in place.
>
> (ibid., pp. 29–30)

When one is a part of this elevated and prioritized group, one does not have the naturally occurring capacity to reflect upon the ingrained beliefs and assumptions inherent within the context of that group. Recently, I asked a practicing religious patient who is in analysis with me about his perspective on an issue that could be seen as a conflict within his belief system. He answered, 'I don't have a personal belief or view about this, it just is'. Here lives the entanglement of the cultural and the personal. When one grows up steeped in belief systems that are supported by cultural structures of authority and power, personal discernment regarding the direct impact (beneficial or harmful) of such belief systems can be like a most challenging knot. As my patient said, 'it just is'.

White body supremacy trauma is the inherited unconscious and unrecognized somatic, familial, and cultural impacts that manifest as *dirty pain*. Menakem describes dirty pain as, 'avoidance, blame, and denial. When people respond from their most wounded parts, become cruel or violent, or physically or emotionally run away. They also create more of it for themselves' (Menakim 2017, p. 20). He suggests, 'if it [white body supremacy trauma] gets transmitted and compounded through multiple families and generations, it can start to look like culture' (ibid., p. 30). Jung speaks to this in his articulation of an activated and complexed archetype saying,

> But if it is a question of a general incompatibility or an otherwise injurious condition productive of neuroses in relatively large numbers of individuals, then we must assume the presence of constellated archetypes since neuroses are in most cases not just private concerns, but social phenomena, we must assume that archetypes are constellated in these cases too. The archetype corresponding to the situation is activated, and as a result those explosive and dangerous forces hidden in the archetype come into action, frequently with unpredictable consequences. There is no lunacy people under the domination of an archetype will not fall prey to.
>
> (Jung 1937/1980, para. 98)

In Jungian theory, we have a method to understand this kind of inherited, intergenerational trauma. Taking Jung's understanding and concepts of both complex theory and the collective unconscious, Jungian Analysts Thomas Singer and Samuel Kimbles (2004) put forward the notion of cultural complexes. Building on Joseph Henderson's idea of the cultural unconscious, an interlocutor layer between the collective unconscious and the personal unconscious, a cultural complex can be understood to reside within the space between the personal and the collective. Henderson defines the cultural unconscious as:

> an area of historical memory that lies between the collective unconscious and the manifest pattern of the cultural. It may include both these modalities,

conscious and unconscious, but it has some kind of identity arising from the archetypes of the collective unconscious, which assists in the formation of myth and ritual and also *promotes the process of development in individuals.*
(Henderson 1990, p. 182)

Singer and Kimbles describe how the cultural complex 'exists within the psyche of the collective as a whole and the individual members of the group … and … mostly have to do with trauma, discrimination, feelings of oppression and inferiority at the hands of another offending group' (2004, p. 177). Putting this Jungian concept of the cultural complex with Menakem's work on white body supremacy trauma, we see how culture is mapped out of our personal and collective wounds. These wounds seek to inject a sense of evil and otherness unconsciously experienced within the insider who represents the dominant culture, into the outsider, the *other* outside of majority culture, outside of hegemonic power structures. Once the evil is extracted out of the *insider* (the white-bodied person who holds the dominant cultural power) and injected into the *outsider* (the black-bodied person), the insider seeks to paralyze and silence the *other*, the outsider, to resist a feeling of implication. It is exactly this feeling of implication that would open space for integration.

Witnessing Whiteness: Breaking the Silence

Silence is a defense of the ego complex against the rising tide of affect that has been built up through years of collective and cultural suppression. I see silence as the gatekeeper of emotion. Dirty pain thwarts a working-through of the intergenerational trauma of white body supremacy (Menakem 2017). As Hannah Zeavin says, 'Neutrality is also protective … it confers the power on psychoanalysis to sit outside time, place, politics, and history' (Zeavin 2021, p. 8).

Much of our work as analysts falls within the phenomenon of bearing witness. We stand witness to the vicissitudes of our patients' experiences, past and present, as well as their fantasies. The early childhood trauma that was survived and is now being related to, the horrific experience of personal and social wounding, the debilitating depressions and psychotic episodes, the joy, the laughter, the slow growth of consciousness that inches its way around and around, backward, and forward, *to*-ing and *fro*-ing from the center to the periphery. It is, of course, easier to bear witness to that to which we have had some exposure. It comes more naturally to witness and affirm the aspects of the patient's Self that penetrate the rigidity of their conscious ego when the images, motifs, and dynamics of Self follow a trajectory that is more familiar to the analyst. However, when confronted with images that are unfamiliar or are perhaps threatening—statements or feelings that arise from the patient that challenge our own way(s) of knowing and being—it is all too common to allow the unfamiliarity to go unacknowledged. When unacknowledged feeling states or images emerge but are not related to, they remain in unconscious suspension. We may speak of this suspension as a type of paralysis that puts unacknowledged feelings at risk of erasure. Comments that may prick something within us analysts, that we cannot understand or that we feel ashamed of, fall by the wayside and are not picked-up for play, for discussion, or for relating.

I often hear Jungian analysts uphold the concept of analytic abstinence. This is an analytic stance that claims neutrality on the side of the analyst born out of one's own process of individuation through one's own long-term personal analysis. It is taught, the role of the analyst is to remain neutral, free of judgment, engaging with the symbols that arise in the psychic process of the patient without an agenda, not to proselytize, convert, exhort, judge, or correct the analysand's behavior from one's own personal stance. This is, in one major way, what often distinguishes analysis from therapy. The analyst listens to the patient's life story, learning of the earliest encounters with others and self, listening for the patient's own road map coming forth from the Self, that other that is simultaneously personal and transpersonal (Jung 1951/1979).[1] The Jungian Analyst also listens symbolically to the movement and work of psyche within the narrative, symptoms, symbols, and relationships of the analysand. This kind of listening and reflecting with the analysand focuses the work on the contents of the unconscious expressed in dreams, enactments, repetitions, and the intersubjective relationship or the transference and counter-transference dynamics between analyst and analysand. As Jungian Analysts, we are encouraged to *follow psyche*, meaning, to follow the transpersonal energetic movement that arises in the patients dreams and unconscious contents. Our job is to work with the images psyche presents to and within the patient and to translate these images, symbolically allowing these images to speak their own truth, their own story to the life of the patient.

The training for the analyst is specific, deep, and personal. What is required first and foremost, is a rigorous ongoing relationship with one's own unconscious process. Second of importance is a wide breadth of knowledge of mythology and different symbol systems that might come up within the unconscious of the patient that might be unfamiliar to the analyst. What is equally important to this second tenet is a working knowledge of diverse cultures and their religious or spiritual systems, worldviews, and mythological tropes.

Jung himself placed a high value on traveling the world and immersing himself in a variety of cultures, studying their religious systems, cultural rituals and customs, and their symbolic objects (Jung 1989, pp. 238–84). However, Jung's exploration of the other (external) was in service of his own other (internal) and a byproduct of the white imaginary (Saban 2019). His inquiry had an unfortunate result of appropriation. He was searching the world over, far, and wide, to find a symbol system that would help him map out his unique view of psyche and psychic process and transformation. In addition, he was taking his own method and looking for ways in which various cultures affirmed the relevance of his method (Brewster 2017, 2020). From *Gnosticism* in the texts of the Ancient Near East (Jung 1951/1979, par. 287–346); to typology gleaned from the European philosophers, poets and writers (Jung 1921/1976); to the ancient Chinese Taoist text, the *Secret of the Golden Flower* (Jung 1929/1970); and then finally to his work with the late medieval tradition of *Alchemy* (1955/1977), Jung was looking for a symbol system that reflected what *he* experienced as psychic process both within himself and within the patients, nearly all white Europeans, with whom he worked and eventually birthed the unique branch of psychoanalysis that became known as Analytical Psychology.

It was through his engagement and experiential research in other cultures and with a plethora of diverse texts that he penned the concept of the collective unconscious (Jung 1937/1980, para. 88). The uniqueness, and I would argue relevance, of Jungian psychology lies within Jung's notion that psyche and psychological process include the collective in addition to the personal unconscious. For Jung, psychological development within the individual is limited when kept within the frame of the personal unconscious. Whereas in the personal unconscious we find all those contents that have been forgotten or, due to the demands of one's own upbringing and development, have been repressed (Jung 1916/1972, para. 218). Within the collective unconscious live all those contents that have not yet been known to consciousness (Jung 1937/1980, para. 90). These contents, Jung argues, are timeless and shared between all cultures and people groups. As he describes it,

> the unconscious, as the totality of all archetypes, is the deposit of all human experience right back to its remotest beginnings. Not, indeed, a dead deposit, a sort of abandoned rubbish heap, but a living system of actions and aptitudes that determine the individual's life in invisible ways—all the more effective because invisible. It is not a gigantic historical prejudice, so to speak, an a priori historical condition; but it is also the source of all instincts, for the archetypes are simply the forms which the instincts assume.
>
> (Jung 1931/1975, para. 339)

I argue that we can understand white body supremacy as an archetypal experience of the Other, through Jung's notion of the collective unconscious and the objectivity of psyche. Ann Ulanov expands on Jung's notion by saying,

> psyche exists prior to and independently of consciousness, which emerges from it. Paradoxically, psyche is an objective reality which we are accustomed to think of as existing within us or as being a function of our subjective consciousness, but which, in fact, acts in relation to us as an "other."
>
> (Ulanov 1971, p. 18)

Jung argued that the collective unconscious is a

> second psychic system of a collective, universal, and impersonal nature which is identical in all individuals ... is inherited ... and consists of pre-existent forms, the archetypes, which can only become conscious second-arily and which give definite form to certain psychic contents.
>
> (Jung 1937/1980, para. 90)

I believe we can understand white supremacy as a definite form of a psychic content that exists in all individuals, namely, the psychic content of the *Other*. *Other*, I define, as that which is *not-me*. "Me" is understood here as that which is defined as right, good, acceptable, and "normal" by dominant culture. That which is *not-me* is that which is not right, not acceptable, out of the bounds of normal, unknown, alien, foreign.[2] What Jung adds to the rich history of the study of the other is his notion of the self, the other that confronts us within, a transpersonal control point (Jung 1953, para. 217) or self-representations of unconscious develop-ments (ibid., para. 216), that which is in us but bigger than us, beyond the personal yet confronting us personally, bringing in that which has never before been in.

Resmaa Menakem warns his readers before entering his book, *My Grandmother's Hands: Racialized Trauma and the Pathway to Mending our Hearts and Bodies* (2017),

> If you are convinced that ending white supremacy begins with social and political action, do not read this book unless you are willing to be challenged. We need to begin with the healing of trauma—in dark-skinned bodies, light-skinned bodies, our neighborhoods and communities, and the law enforcement profession. Social and political actions are essential, but they need to be part of a larger strategy of healing, justice, and creating room for growth in traumatized flesh-and-blood bodies.
>
> (Menakem 2017, p. ix)

Menakem puts forth a way of understanding white body supremacy through the lens of trauma theory. He contends,

> White-body supremacy is always functioning in our bodies. It operates in our thinking brains, in our assumptions, expectations and mental short-cuts. It operates in our muscles and nervous systems, where it routinely creates constriction. But it operates most powerfully in our lizard brains. Our lizard brain cannot think. It is reflexively protective, and it is strong. It loves whatever it feels will keep us safe, and it fears and hates whatever it feels will do us harm.
>
> (Menakim 2017, p. 6)

I hear this through Jung's understanding of the archetypes of the collective unconscious, what he calls:

> ancient images restored to life by the primitive, analogical mode of thinking peculiar to dreams. It is not a question of inherited ideas, but of inherited thought-patterns ... the unconscious contains not only personal, but also impersonal collective components in the form of inherited categories or archetypes.
>
> (Jung 1916/1972, para. 220)

Holding Menakem's notion of white body supremacy trauma with Jung's notion of the collective unconscious as inherited thought-patterns, I turn now to the concept of the implicated subject, proffered by Michael Rothberg (2019). Together, these three concepts begin to speak to the silence, or *dirty pain*, that has been historically perpetuated within white dominant spaces and culture. Before turning fully to Rothberg, I will bring this conversation more intimately into the world of Jungian Analysis and Jungian and broader psychoanalytic learning and training communities.

Donald Moss, faculty, and psychoanalyst with the New York Psychoanalytic Institute, contends, in his article 'On Having Whiteness' (2020), that whiteness 'opportunistically attaches to any psychic structure that maps self and object vertically. These vertical planes are ubiquitous and as such provide an abundance of potential host receptors for Parasitic Whiteness' (p. 359). He describes the vertical planes along six different lines, each of which delineate inner and outer, or inside and outside, with the good being inside and the bad being outside. He continues,

> Along each of these vertical planes, subject–object relations are defined by power and grounded in the fantasy of sovereignty. And along each of these vertical planes, safety, satisfaction, and pleasure are necessarily fragile and contingent. Everything I have, everything I am, can be lost: my strength turned to abjection, my inclusion to exile, my calm to terror.
>
> (Moss 2020, p. 360)

The publication of Moss's article resulted in him receiving numerous death threats from the alt-right. From his psychoanalytic colleagues and the liberal left he was written off as writing about a topic that did not have a place within the psychoanalytic field. In her recent article, 'Unfree Association' (2022), his stepdaughter Hannah Zeavin writes that Moss was seen as a discipline traitor. The psychoanalytic community felt him to be making race and racism a central node of the psyche. She relates, 'He got into trouble with his peers not for how he addressed whiteness, per se, but for violating the white analytic tradition of not addressing it at all' (p. 13).

Since June 2020, businesses, institutes of higher education, and organizations of all kinds have been asked to deeply examine every aspect of their practices for the ways in which they have been implicitly aligned with white supremacy in their business practices. When bringing this issue into the psychoanalytic space, it is immediately met with either caution or suspicion. The guild states that this kind of work belongs not in the psychoanalytic space where we attempt to achieve neutrality. The work—meaning consciousness around the ways in which whiteness or white body supremacy trauma infect and affect each and every person, as the argument goes—is not necessarily relevant when it comes to the analytic ethic of the analytic dyad. If we are under the ethic of neutrality, our job as analyst is not to bring our "political, social, or religious" views into the analytic container. However, I contend that the reality of trauma of white supremacy on all bodies is neither a political nor a social issue. White supremacy trauma lives in the collective unconscious. It is archetypal in nature. We know of its impact through the body.

The backlash from the right and the left to psychoanalyst Donald Moss's paper highlights the intensity of the racial complex that, I argue, is better understood as an archetype of the collective unconscious. It is beyond the personal yet must be addressed at the personal level. Moss describes whiteness as 'a condition one first acquires and then *has*—a malignant, parasitic-like condition to which "white" people have a particular susceptibility'. He states, 'Whiteness originates not in innocence but in entitlement' (Moss 2020, p. 4).

This condition described by Moss is foundational. It generates characteristic ways of being in one's body, in one's mind, and in the world. Parasitic Whiteness renders its hosts' appetites voracious, insatiable, and perverse. These deformed appetites particularly target nonwhite peoples. Once established, these appetites are nearly impossible to eliminate. With this definition in mind, we return to the image of Missy thrusting Chris into *the sunken place* and the image of the silent but voraciously hungry white bidders vying for Chris's body (Peele 2017). Effective treatment consists of a combination of psychic and social-historical interventions, argues Moss. In concert with Moss, I argue that the mutative agent that allows for effective treatment here is found in the feeling function and in the body. What neutrality allows for is the primacy of the experience of the Other with whom we work. However, neutrality also has a protective function. It allows the analyst to remain on the outside, not to be taken in or drowned by the patient's suffering or experiences. Another outcome of neutrality, I argue, is a defense against the intimacy that the horror of the other brings and evokes within ourselves, silencing the felt impact of one's own implication (Rothberg 2019, p. 80).

Implicated Subjects: A New Analytic Ethic Speaking to Parasitic Whiteness

In 'After the Catastrophe' (1945), written after WWI and just at the cusp of WWII, Jung writes:

since no man lives within his own psychic sphere like a snail in its shell, separated from everybody else, but is connected with his fellow-men by his unconscious humanity, no crime can ever be what it appears to our consciousness to be: an isolated psychic happening.

(Jung 1945/1964, para. 408)

In this article he relates collective guilt to a state of magical uncleanness. He expands further,

It is a fact that cannot be denied: the wickedness of others becomes our own wickedness because it kindles something evil in our own hearts. The murder has been suffered by everyone, and everyone has committed it; lured by the irresistible fascination of evil, we have all made this collective psychic murder possible; and the closer we were to it the better we could see, the greater our guilt. In this way we are unavoidably drawn into the uncleanness of evil, no matter what our conscious attitude may be.

(Jung 1945/1964, para. 408)

Jung is describing what Michael Rothberg (2019) articulates as the implicated subject. In Rothberg's articulation, building on Hannah Arendt's (2003) work around collective responsibility, he proposes to move beyond the binary of victim and perpetrator to offer a third way. In the binary of victim and perpetrator, one can find a way to silence the feelings that arise from owning one's own participation in collective harm. While one may not be complicit in evil done to others, meaning the direct perpetrators of harm, one may be implicitly involved. Knowing about horrors and remaining silent in the face of them, implicates one in the perpetuation of harm. Rothberg defines implicated subjects:

[As those who] Occupy positions aligned with power and privilege without being themselves direct agents of harm; they contribute to, inhabit, inherit, or benefit from regimes of domination but do not originate or control such regimes. An implicated subject is neither a victim nor a perpetrator, but rather a participant in histories and social formations that generate the positions of victim and perpetrator, and yet in which most people do not occupy such clear-cut roles ... implicated subjects help propagate the legacies of historical violence and prop up the structures of inequality that mar the present.

(Rothberg 2019, pp. 1–2)

Individuation is the process of establishing a robust and vital relationship between the ego and the Self or between consciousness and unconscious contents and process. I suggest that a crucial aspect of the analytic work is to become conscious of how white body supremacy trauma silences and pushes the effects and affects upon all bodies further into the unconscious. A way for white analysts and majority white training institutes to begin bringing consciousness to this real aspect of our American collective is by *feeling into* (rather than thinking about) our own implicated subjectivity on a personal level. For thinking about, and creating theories that help us understand cognitively, allows us to stay on the outside of the horror. Feeling into penetrates us right at the core, bringing us into the center of the horror.

How do white clinicians hear and address the racial complex when it comes into treatment? What about when it enters as a derivative, indirectly? This ultimately depends upon our capacity to hear and a certain ego strength to allow for the penetration of what has before been frozen, paralyzed, and eradicated from consciousness. Rothberg states, 'Implication emerges from the ongoing, uneven, and destabilizing intrusion of irrevocable pasts into the unredeemed present' (Rothberg 2019, p. 9). We cannot hear if we are not aware of it in ourselves first. Jung himself critiques the notion of a personal psychology that remains silently neutral when he says,

> Nevertheless, a purely personalistic psychology, by reducing everything to personal causes, tries its level best to deny the existence of archetypal motifs and even seeks to destroy them by personal analysis. I consider this a rather dangerous procedure which cannot be justified medically … Can we not see how a whole nation is reviving an archaic symbol, yes, even archaic religious forms and how this mass emotion is influencing and revolutionizing the life of the individual in a catastrophic manner? The man of the past is alive in us today to a degree undreamt of before the war, and in the last analysis what is the fate of great nations but a summation of the psychic changes in individuals?
>
> (Jung 1937/1980, para. 97)

A white patient comments on a difficult relationship with her Black friend and roommate:

> '*M* just hates me. She doesn't treat me with any kindness or love. She always assumes the worst of me. *M* begrudges me because I get what I ask for, but I only get what I ask for because I actually ask. She never asks or advocates for herself!'

This is not the first time my patient, whom I will call Alice has come to session activated and highly dysregulated regarding her relationship with her Black roommate. In inquiring further about what she meant when she said her roommate 'never asks or advocates for herself', my white patient, Alice, shared several examples that included asking a salesperson for a different item and asking a restaurant server for a different seat. But the incident she was highlighting specifically was of her call to a hotel to request a later check-out time due to a need to depart later than previously expected. She was perplexed as to how a simple phone call would be difficult for her Black friend, given it was not in person. Surely, Alice thought, *M* would not have any issues arise due to her ethnicity or skin color through a phone exchange. Skin color cannot be seen over the phone, my patient remarks.

In the split second of this exchange, my own mind and body had an immediate response to this comment. Does Alice realize the privilege that comes with being white? Does she realize the ease with which she takes for granted how simple such a question, such as wanting to check out late from a hotel, has been throughout her life? There is an underlying assumption of: 'I see what I want, I can ask for it, and it will, more than likely, be given to me'. It does not cross the mind of the white subject that if something is not granted, it is due to the color of her skin, her accent, tone of voice, the way she phrases a question or comment that lands in the receiver as a threat. This threat is not due to anything other than the unconscious complex that gets activated and ignites a whole history of toxic racialized relations in our country. As I sorted through all these questions and thoughts and how to address them analytically, I felt both implored to speak and paralyzed to speak. I felt my own ease in not speaking, the familiar pull toward silence. I wrestled to bring myself out of my own paralysis, attempting to speak to the difficulties of power and privilege. I, simultaneously, sought to deter from abusing my own privilege as the doctor.

What is the analytic move? How do I work with this racialized complex in a way that opens up rather than shuts down? What is the role of the analyst in addressing systemic racism and how it shows up within the racial complex in the analytic vase? How do I work to help this patient see the underlying racialized assumptions afforded by the privilege granted by her white skin and her own upbringing as I struggle to see the privilege afforded to me that allows me to stay silent? Many white analysts will claim this is not the task of the analyst. During my many years of analytic training, I was not taught to engage dynamics of systemic racism. Often, I do not I feel equipped to work with the racial complex, given the activation of my own racialized complex in such moments. How do I reflect on what has been said without evoking the shame that so quickly creates an impasse?

Rothberg articulates the difference between genealogical implication and structural implication. Rothberg suggests that genealogical implication (e.g., being a literal descendent of a slave owner) is intimate, yet diffuse. Structural implication is diffuse, yet intimate.

> In the case of structural implication there may not be an intimate link to the history of slavery; my connection to the past is discontinuous and diffuse. Out of the diffusion, however, comes an even more intimate determination than the one that follows from (mere) genealogical implication: my very subjectivity as a social being derives from the impersonal structures that surround and support me ... although diffuse, such determinations create us:

subjects occupy a differential position at the intersection of impersonal forces that nevertheless make them who they are.

(Rothberg 2019, p. 79)

Stumbling toward the intimacy found in my own implication with my patient, I found myself saying, 'Isn't it amazing how easy it seems to be for us white women to ask for what it is we want or need without having to be concerned with how the other will perceive us because of the color of our skin or tone of our voice?' She quickly retorts, 'Well, this was a phone call so she wouldn't even have had to worry about the color of her skin'. I felt her close off and shut down. We were in the territory of the complex. In this territory, the patient feels a threat that nears annihilation. I felt the territory we were in palpably in my body. I, myself, felt silenced and strangulated. It is not unlike any other moment when working with a complex: The delicate dance between bringing consciousness to the moment to allow the patient to see more deeply and metabolize the feelings of the complex. This work aims at widening the ego capacity to tolerate dissonance and difficulty to reclaim projections and create more room within the collective. With this racial complex constellating within and between this white patient and her white analyst, it felt as though we were in a minefield. The risk of annihilation hung on every breath.

Perhaps the moment was missed, the intervention was dodged. Likely by us both. I have often been asked by Black, frustrated colleagues and friends why I handhold my white colleagues and white patients regarding the enactment of the racial complex?

Since the murder of George Floyd ignited (another) national reckoning, I have been a part of many analytic circles, groups, classes, institutions, and communities who have been grappling with the analytic response and responsibility to what has been the collective unconscious racial complex within the United States for over 400 years. We know that the story goes back further. The year 1619 is our beginning point, here, on this soil. In these past two years I have heard many different perspectives. There are some communities addressing this horror more directly, perhaps more consciously, within their training curriculum and institutes.

It is my view that the Jungian paradigm offers a nuanced theoretical model to help understand how systematic and systematized racism exist and are unconsciously perpetuated. It is a model that helps us understand the problem of evil. Less discussed, less nuanced, less clear is how to address this problem in the analytic endeavor, both within the analytic vase and in the collective. I have heard it said over and over within the Jungian community that we cannot go where the patient is not ready to go. Said another way, we must follow psyche's trajectory within the patient. I have heard this explained a variety of different ways. Once it was explained that if someone drinks a six-pack of beer nightly but never brings this up as a psychological problem within the treatment, it is clearly not a problem for this person; therefore, the analyst is not to explore this image in the analysis unless the patient starts to indicate he himself feels a conflict within himself around this behavior. This example points to a Jungian perspective that our work is amoral, uninvolved with addressing right and wrong, good, and bad. The amoral psyche's only agenda is in its relation to Self.

I argue that our hegemonic silence as a predominately white and western psychological school of thought and practice perpetuates an aspect of archetypal evil bound up in the concept of the other. The antidote to hegemonic silence is found in recognizing that we are *implicated subjects*, allowing this to penetrate our feeling. As analytical psychologists, we are implicated by the histories into which we have been born and the histories in which we have been rooted.

> Psychological collective guilt is a tragic fate. It hits everybody, just and unjust alike, everybody who was anywhere near the place where the terrible thing happened. Naturally no reasonable and conscientious person will lightly turn collective into individual guilt by holding the individual responsible without giving him a hearing. He will know enough to distinguish between the individually guilty and the merely collectively guilty. But how many people are either reasonable or conscientious, and how many take the trouble to become so?
>
> (Jung 1945/1964, para. 405)

Jung continues:

> the wickedness of others becomes our own wickedness because it kindles something evil in our own hearts. The murder has been suffered by everyone, and everyone has committed it; lured by the irresistible fascination of evil, we have all made this collective psychic murder possible; and the closer we were to it the better we could see, the greater our guilt. In this way we are unavoidably drawn into the uncleanness of evil, no matter what our conscious attitude may be.
>
> (Jung 1945/1964, para. 408)

It is my conviction that it is an analytic necessity and my ethical responsibility as a Jungian psychoanalyst, to work toward my own understanding and to feel my implication in the history of racism in our country. This work is not political or ideological. Rather, this work is the only way to stop perpetuating the dirty pain of silence and paralysis enacted within the analytic vase. Investigative journalist Nikole Hannah-Jones (Klein 2021) talks about how we are not responsible for our ancestors, but that we are responsible for what we know now and for continually learning about the effects of our ancestors' choices upon us today. We are also charged to respond to this knowing. This article is a response to this knowing.

Notes

1 I employ Jung's notion of the Self here, as opposed to the notion of the self used within the school of Self psychology.
2 Given the limits of this chapter, I do not have the space to provide a more thorough review of the concept of the other as articulated in fields of phenomenology and philosophy which date back to the late 1700s and the concepts first articulated by Hegel, Husserl, de Beauvoir, and later by psychoanalysts and ethicists Lacan and Levinas, Laing, and the more contemporary Kearney. However, there is a rich field of study and research around this psychic fact and experience of "the other."

References

Arendt, H. (2003). "Collective Responsibility", in *Responsibility and Judgment*, ed. Jerome Kohn. New York: Schocken.

Bellot, G. (2021). "How Black Horror Became America's Most Powerful Cinematic Genre". *The New York Times Style Magazine*. https://www.nytimes.com/2021/11/10/t-magazine/black-horror-films-get-out.html.

Brewster, F. (2020). *The Racial Complex*. New York: Routledge.

Brewster, F. (2017). *African Americans and Jungian Psychology: Leaving the Shadows*. New York: Taylor & Francis.

DiAngelo, R. (2018). *White Fragility*. Boston, MA: Beacon Press.

Henderson, J. (1990). "The Cultural Unconscious". *Shadow and Self*. Silmette, IL: Chiron Publications.

Jung, C.G. (1916/1972). "The Relation between the Ego and the Unconscious". *CW* 7.

Jung, C.G. (1921/1976). *Psychological Types. CW* 6.

Jung, C.G. (1929/1970). "Commentary on 'The Secret of the Golden Flower'". *CW 13*.

Jung, C.G. (1931/1975). "The Structure of the Psyche". *CW* 8. Princeton: Princeton University Press.

Jung, C.G. (1937/1980). 'The Concept of the Collective Unconscious'. *CW 9i*.

Jung, C.G. (1945/1964). "After the Catastrophe". *CW 10*.

Jung, C.G. (1951/1979). "The Self", *CW* 9ii.

Jung, C.G. (1953/1972). "The Personal and the Collective Unconscious". *CW 7*.

Jung, C.G. (1955/1977). *Mysterium Coniunctionis. CW* 14.

Jung, C.G. (1989). *Memories, Dreams, Reflections*. New York: Vintage Books Edition.

Iati, M. (2021). "What is Critical Race Theory and Why do Republicans Want to Ban it in Schools? *The Washington Post*, 29 May. https://www.washingtonpost.com/education/2021/05/29/critical-race-theory-bans-schools/

Klein, E. (2021). Podcast. "What's Really Behind the 1619 Backlash? An Interview with Ta-Nehisi Coates and Nikole Hannah-Jones". *The New York Times*. https://www.nytimes.com/2021/07/30/opinion/ezra-klein-podcast-ta-nehisi-coates-nikole-hannah-jones.html

Mills, C. (1997). *The Racial Contract*. New York: Cornell University Press.

Menakem, R. (2017). *My Grandmother's Hands: Racialized Trauma and the Pathway to Mending Our Hearts and Bodies*. Las Vegas, NV: Central Recovery Press.

Morgan, H. (2021). *The Work of Whiteness: A Psychoanalytic Perspective*. Routledge: New York.

Moss, D. (2020). "On Having Whiteness". *Journal of the American Psychoanalytic Association*, 69, 2, 355–371.

Peale, J. (2017). *Get Out*.

Rankine, C. & Loffreda, B. (2015). *The Racial Imaginary: Writers on Race in the Life of the Mind*. New York: Fence Books.

Rothberg, M. (2019). *The Implicated Subject: Beyond Victims and Perpetrators*. Stanford: Stanford University Press.

Saban, M. (2019). *'Two Souls Alas' Jungs Two Personalities and the Making of Analytical Psychology*. Asheville, NC: Chiron Publications.

Sheehi, L. & Sheehi, S. (2021). *Psychoanalysis Under Occupation: Practicing Resistance in Palestine*. New York: Taylor and Francis.

Singer, T. & Kimbles, S. (2004). "Emerging Theory of Cultural Complexes". *Analytical Psychology*. London & New York: Routledge.

Ulanov, A.B. (1971). *The Feminine in Jungian Psychology and in Christian Theology*. Evanston: Northwestern University Press.

Zeavin, H. (2022). "Unfree Associations: Parasitic Whiteness on and off the Couch". *N+1 Magazine*. Spring, 42: *Vanishing Act*.

Chapter 8

Reparative Transgression
A psychoanalytic institute reckons – and does not reckon – with its own racism

Sarah J. Braun

Addressing and making reparations for the harm of racism is a task that can never be completed. This is cause for both despair and hope: despair, because on the individual and collective levels we will never rid ourselves of racism, and we will never repair all of the harm that has been caused because of it; and hope, because we always have the opportunity to contribute to the work that so urgently needs to be done.

In the summer of 2020 Black Lives Matter rose more forcefully than ever from the ashes of generations lost to and violated by systemic racism. As I stood in Philadelphia, in the presence of the human river of protestors, I was flooded by both hope and despair. I felt sickened by the realization that many of those gathered to give voice to the outrage were those most likely to be harmed by the virus in our midst, present in the necessary protest we had come to join. As a psychoanalyst and physician, I feared that viral exposure at the protests would result in more suffering and death in communities already most harmed by institutional racism and injustice. I am grateful that I was wrong.

This is one example of psychic energy manifesting collectively, embodying fierceness both in the service of greater life *and* in the service of destruction, both fulfilling and destroying possibilities by crossing boundaries deemed taboo. When greater life and wholeness, rather than greater destruction, arises from such a process, I have come to name it *redemptive transgression*. A central challenge as psychoanalysts is to discern with our patients (to the extent that it is possible) whether a given potential transgression is redemptive or not. When and how do we know?

In our current collective field, *reparative transgression* more closely captures a related process at work. In our society's reckoning—and *not* reckoning—more substantially with the reality of our country's founding and growth on the backs and blood of enslaved and original people, the possibility of making both concrete and symbolic reparation for past harms has been foregrounded. Psychoanalytic institutes have an analogous responsibility to address more fully and make reparations for our exclusion and erasure of Black and Brown analysands, candidates and analysts by our past

DOI: 10.4324/9781003311447-9

dismissiveness, inadequate acknowledgement and lack of consistency in explicitly addressing racism and other destructive elements in our training.[1] Acknowledging the harm that theory and writings we value have inflicted can register to some as destructively transgressive, diminishing the value of our 'ancestors'; yet it mirrors, on a group level, Jung's recognition that "[e]very individual needs revolution, inner division, overthrow of the existing order, and renewal" (Jung 1917/1972, p. 5).

A different version of this kind of renewal occurred in the 1990s, in psychoanalytic communities. *Lingering Shadows: Jungians, Freudians, and Anti-Semitism* (Maidenbaum & Martin 1991) was published shortly before I began my analytic training. As a practicing Jew, I experienced the publication and existence of this book, and the conference from which it emerged, as implicitly welcoming, although, poorly versed in Jung as I was, I had been only vaguely aware of his anti-Semitism and how it manifested in his writings. 'Why would you train as a Jungian psychoanalyst? He was an anti-Semite!' was a question asked/accusation made of me at times by other Jews, marked like me by the Holocaust of the Second World War. A question which troubled me and to which I had no adequate response.

As I continued in training and in psychoanalytic practice, I appreciated more deeply the significance of the Jungian community's acknowledgment and exploration of Jung's anti-Semitism, including the unresolved, and unresolvable, questions that remain regarding the totality of Jung's conscious and unconscious attitude towards Jews, as well as the attitudes of those who were influenced by Jung and his writings. I also have valued having an identifiable source that I could draw on to respond to the question that so unsettled me. It is a testament to the efforts of the psychoanalytic community's public grappling with Jung's anti-Semitism that the thesis I wrote as part of the culmination of my analytic training was an examination of archetypal and clinical correspondences of the Jewish ritual of *Havdalah*, which marks the transition between the Jewish sabbath and secular week. It is even more telling that I did not register any hesitation in pursuing this material which was of great personal meaning for me.

Black and Brown analysands, candidates, and analysts—and all whose identities have been either explicitly or implicitly minimized, denigrated, infantilized, or demonized in Jung's writings and teaching, or, in the work of other members of the analytical psychology community—deserve to have such sources, and to experience as well the kind of welcoming attitude from which I and other Jewish analysands, candidates, and analysts have benefited. The reality that the cultural complex around racism is brutal and powerful in ways that to a certain extent overlap with (and in other ways are utterly distinct from) that which is activated around anti-Semitism intensifies the necessity of this undertaking in our community.

I read it as life-giving to hold both the value of Jung's profound awarenesses and contributions along with the harm caused by his failings, conscious and otherwise. This also applies to our own contributions and failings as individuals and as psychoanalytic institutes and communities. As we take responsibility for harm, what reparations are called for? Can we make them without inflicting more harm because of our 'dumb fish' unawareness?[2] In the spirit of furthering consciousness by reflection, I use analytical psychology methods, drawing on transgressions and reparations in rituals associated with the Jewish holiday of Passover to consider archetypal energies underlying my personal experience of the attempts our institute has made as we strive to be aware of and make space for what and whom we have excluded.

This piece is neither a critique of how our institute has (and has not) responded to this call for greater consciousness, nor a criticism of any individuals or groups within our institute. It is rather, one white Jewish analyst's attempt to describe and reflect on some of the archetypal dynamics at work in this liminal moment as they manifest in one institute, and in my individual psyche.

Several significant works have been published in our psychoanalytic community which speak to the intergenerational transmission of group trauma, including racism (Kimbles 2014), and to racism in Jung's writings and in aspects of theory underlying analytical psychology (Adams 1996; Brewster 2017, 2020; Morgan 2021; Brewster & Morgan 2022). However, as Carter (2021) has enunciated, our teaching of candidates and the way we work with theoretical and clinical material in our learning community do not yet reflect the degree of integration of these understandings that provides Black and Brown members (and potential members) of our community a genuinely adequate sense of having a full voice and place at the table.

As a Jungian analyst, I had been involved with the Jungian Psychoanalytic Association (JPA) only peripherally since it was founded (2004), a few years after I had finished my analytic training at the C. G. Jung Institute of New York (CGJINY). I chose to support the creation of the JPA because most (although not all) of the analysts whom I knew best—those with whom I had gone through training and those who had been my teachers and supervisors—were choosing to do the same. Recently graduated, and living and practicing in Philadelphia, I joined the Philadelphia Association of Jungian Analysts, where I became part of the analyst faculty for the seminar and candidate training program. I was not active in teaching or serving on committees in New York, and I did not directly witness or experience the conversations and dynamics that engendered the JPA. My rudimentary understanding was that there was an intention for less scrutiny of candidates' personal psyches, as well as for a more expansive approach to the teaching of analytical psychology than existed in the institute in which I had trained. I also understood that the JPA intended to create a community that would regularly bring together analyst members and candidates to share in learning from each other and from invited speakers. Over the following 20 years, before the COVID pandemic that descended in 2020, my relationship with the JPA consisted of following email communications sent to analyst members, as well as personal and professional relationships within the membership body.

Whatever the impetus was for the creation of the JPA, it was, by definition, transgressively created, involving a crossing of the previously held boundary of the CGJINY and a rupture in what had been a single community. Like many transgressions, it has had both destructive and life-giving consequences. I will return to reflections on some of these consequences later in this chapter.

I have been at the boundary of the JPA, part in and part out, since its inception. The Biblical Hebrew word *ivri* refers to a member of the people who left Egypt and became the Jewish people. Its literal meaning is 'one who crosses (a boundary)'. It captures many aspects of my experience: as a psychiatrist in a largely non-medical psychoanalytic community; as a member of two different Jungian psychoanalytic communities; and, as a Jew whose religious practice and sacred calendar at times collides with/sets me apart from the rhythms and timing of our country's ostensibly secular but nonetheless substantially Christian calendar. When do I cross over the boundary of my religious observance in the service of engagement with and contributing to the work of the larger communities that matter to me? When do I hold back from that crossing over? How can I honor the complexity of both of these valued, yet, at times colliding/opposed, aspects of my identity? While I do not attribute this boundary-straddling aspect of my psyche to being Jewish *per se*, I nonetheless recognize the presence of that energy, and appreciate that it contributes to the position I have in relationship to our institute's efforts (and the position aspects of my psyche have to being 'in' or 'out').

I experienced the publication of Christopher Carter's paper in the *Journal of Analytical Psychology* (Carter 2021) and Tiffany Houck's initiation of a group to take up our own racism as white analysts and candidates as a 'second-person call' (Darwall 2006) that brought me further into the JPA. Participating as an 'implicated subject' (Rothberg 2019) in the group that responded to this invitation has been life-giving and excruciating. The latter in keeping with what DiAngelo (2018) names 'white fragility'.[3] My particular mortification has been a striking capacity for acute stupidity, in which I forget or mis-reference the names and works of people of color, and my subjective experience of anxiety in speaking in the group, encouraging as I have found the spirit of the group, and as uncharacteristic as that is for me generally to feel.

My voids and errors reflect the earliest version of racism that I grew up with: One in which, in the middle-class Southern California world of my childhood, in the public schools I attended I had no Black classmates until high school, and I was astonishingly blind to the absence of people of color at the public beaches we enjoyed. While I hope I would have registered it if there were explicitly racist signs prohibiting people of color from those schools or beaches—signs which I knew existed in the South, and which horrified and enraged me—I was oblivious at the time to the presence of the deep and broad forces that bleached the narrow slice of the world that I inhabited.

Being raised in a practicing Jewish family both sensitized me to and insulated me from recognizing and taking responsibility for racism. Our synagogue community was vocal and active in aspects of the American civil rights movement of the 1960s and 1970s; our rabbi had been active in supporting Martin Luther King, Jr., along with Rabbi Abraham Joshua Heschel, and he consistently challenged us to do more to take on the violence and inequities in our society. He also established an organization to honor 'righteous Gentiles', people in the second World War who risked their own safety to protect Jews from persecution and death at the hands of the Nazis. Yet then, even more than now, Judaism was an overwhelmingly white religion, one in which being a member is still at its core based on being the direct descendant of a Jewish parent. Although the Jewish communities I am part of now have an increasing presence of members of color, that profoundly formative domain of my life continues to be predominately white.

Turning to the anxiety, and, the experience of holding back that I wrestle with as part of the JPA group that is attending to our own racism and white privilege, I find another thread woven in. My understanding from conversations over the years with JPA analysts and candidates is that despite holding an intention to foster a spirit of open exchange of ideas and perspectives, the JPA has been experienced by a number of participants as a community in which it can feel transgressively risky to engage authentically. These participants have felt responded to in a hostile or dismissive manner when putting forward perspectives that may challenge or be different from what is seen as aligned with the versions of analytical psychology held to be most valuable by senior analysts, whether in certain classes or in discussions in community-wide clinical evenings or colloquia.[4] Some have noted to me that because of these experiences, and the anxiety engendered by the prospect of having such experiences again, they have tended to not contribute to discussions.

The leadership of the JPA over the years has been aware of this dynamic, and has made efforts to address it, and important shifts have occurred. At the same time, as I have become more involved in the JPA, I have directly experienced the presence of an energy that seems to result in many members of this learning community holding back from voicing their thoughts and responses. My engagement in colloquia and clinical evenings has occurred entirely during the time that these activities, because of the risks of the COVID pandemic, have been conducted exclusively virtually. I recognize that this may contribute inhibiting effects on what otherwise might be a freer, more fluid and robust exchange.

While it will never be possible to know conclusively, I sense that the overarching anxiety some have about sharing aloud their ideas and responses with the larger JPA learning community is a haunting presence that accentuates the anxiety that attends addressing racism in particular. It has been my experience that whatever dynamics exist in a group overall—whether destructive or life-giving—tend to intensify in relationship to racism.

I am mindful that in writing this I am likely to be crossing into territory that has been inhabited by the JPA community for much longer than I have been involved. I have tremendous respect and gratitude for the JPA and I value the opportunity to be part of the community. I do not see the JPA as singularly problematic in its dynamics, and I see many ways in which we strive for and are able to embody much that furthers the process of attending to acknowledgment and inclusion. I am certain that there are a multitude of ways this happens of which I am unaware as well. It is in this context that I lift up the difficulties that I have recognized and experienced, in keeping with the spirit of the ancient challenge from the Babylonian Talmud: **'You are not obligated to finish the task but neither are you free to neglect it'** (Cahan 1998, p. 263).

Hesitations and Anxieties

In trying to contribute to this collection of essays, I have felt paralyzed by the tension between the pull to draw from a familiar symbolic world—Jewish traditions, sacred texts, and literature—and the sinking recognition that this only accentuates a voice from the largely white Jewish perspective, and so risks taking up space that could be occupied by exploring analogous traditions, sacred text, and literature of cultures of color. Yet this is where I land.

This attempt also evokes a version of 'the anxiety of representation' (Zornberg 2001), the awareness of the risk/certainty that whatever I write will cause unintended harm, by both what I include, and, what I unwittingly omit. White fragility, which I will later explain can be understood as a form of *hametz*, raises its head.

It is with these awarenesses, all incomplete, that I offer an exploration of ways in which certain rituals of the Jewish holiday of Passover characterize some aspects of the archetypal experience of anxiety activated by approaching boundaries that seem dangerous but necessary to cross, and, the paradoxes that arise within the psyche in such circumstances. The specific context of these rituals—their relationship to a narrative of the process of liberation from en-slavement—is evocative of the forces at work in my individual psyche and in my experience as a member of the JPA as we discover how to engage as a community in addressing the racism that exists in our field. This associative web underscores the ethical imperative we have as analysts: To engage fully, not to be paralyzed or held captive by the anxiety or sense of shame in the face of the ways that we as individuals, and, our psychoanalytic community as a whole, have—and have not—reckoned with the racism contained in some of Jung's writings and theory. In doing so, I register a mix of urgency, anxiety, vigilance, despair, paralysis, mortification, relief, gratitude and hope, elements that rise and fall without a final resolution.

Passover: Crossing Boundaries

The holiday of Passover is an annual imaginal re-engagement with a foundational myth of Judaism: the experience of enslavement and the liberation from that oppression. In the mythical imagination of the Hebrew Bible and the rabbinical works of the Talmud and beyond, the identity of the Hebrews as a people entering history ostensibly began at the time of this exodus from Egypt.[5] Occurring in the spring, the holiday is infused with a sense of possibility and renewal, curiosity and celebration, as well as a recognition of the suffering involved in being brutally restricted and controlled. The Hebrew word for Egypt is *Mitzrayim*, the narrow places. Freedom and responsibility are intertwined in the telling, the *Maggid*, of this narrative that lies at the heart of the *Seder* and the *Haggadah* that is its guidebook, the highly participatory, multi-sensory ritual meal at the beginning of the holiday. By including descriptive phrases from the Biblical text as well as Talmudic commentaries, eliciting questioning and explicitly encouraging discussion, the *Maggid* includes and fulfills the instruction that *in every generation, every person is obligated to consider themselves*[6] *as having personally left Egypt*. I will take up several aspects of this ritual meal in sections that follow; however, before doing so, I will consider a ritual that precedes the Seder.

Bedikat Hametz – Seeking out the Forbidden

Less familiar to most people than the Passover Seder is the ritual that directly precedes the beginning of the holiday. On the night *before* the first night of Passover many Jews carry out the ritual of *bedikat hametz*: seeking out leavened food. The primary commandment associated with Passover is to eat *matzah* (unleavened bread) and to *not* eat *hametz* (leavened food). In the Bible, *matzah* figures as the bread that the Hebrews brought in their sudden flight from Egypt and slavery, a departure so abrupt that there was no time for the dough to rise, and when it was baked by the sun, as they carried it on their backs, it was flat and hard. In the language of the *Haggadah*, it is 'the bread of affliction' and 'the bread of poverty', and is one of the three most discussed items on the Seder plate. If it is not discussed, one has not fulfilled the requirements of the Seder; if one does not eat it, one has not fulfilled the primary commandment of the holiday.

By contrast, the eating of *hametz* during Passover carries with it *karet*, considered by many traditional commentators to be the severest consequence in all Jewish law, even harsher than capital punishment. Homiletically, *hametz* is associated with arrogance and pretentiousness—a 'puffed-up' sense of self-importance, selfishness, and, invulnerability. *Karet* is a state of utter excommunication, from both the Jewish community of one's lived life and one's spiritual place in Judaism, for all time. The stakes involved in eating *hametz* during Passover could not be higher.

Bedikat hametz is carried out in the following manner: in the month preceding Passover, traces of *hametz* are removed from one's home, workplace, and, even vehicle. The night before the first Seder, a thorough inspection of one's home and its contents (including drawers, shelves, pockets of one's clothing) is conducted for any crumbs of bread or other food considered *hametz*. After setting aside all the *hametz* that has been found, one places several pieces of *hametz* in various locations in the home. By the light of a single candle, after reciting the blessing for seeking out *hametz*, one takes up a large wooden spoon and a feather and brushes each piece into the spoon, collecting them. One then makes a declaration that 'all leaven or anything leavened which is in my possession, whether I have seen it or not, whether I have observed it or not, whether I have removed it or not, shall be considered nullified and ownerless as the dust of the earth'.

Lynn Gottlieb, a modern woman rabbi evokes an intrapsychic version of the experience:

' ... We light a candle
and search in the listening silence
search the high places
and the low places
inside you
search the attic and the basement
the crevices and crannies
the corners of the unused rooms.
Look in your pockets
and the pockets of those around you
for the traces of Mitzrayim.

Some use a feather
some use a knife
to enter the hard places.
Some destroy Hametz with fire
others throw it to the wind
others toss it to the sea.
Look deep for the Hametz
which still gives you pleasure
and cast it to the burning ... .'
                    (Gottlieb 1983, p. 128)

In this rendering, *Mitzrayim* and *hametz*, like racism, are understood as an inner state of being, not denied or projected on an outer enemy or 'other.'

The following morning, by the light of day, a blessing is made before the gathered *hametz* is burnt and the declaration is made again. Gottlieb frames the inner process this way:

' ... When the looking is done
we say:

All that rises up bitter
All that rises up prideful
All that rises up in old ways no longer fruitful
All Hametz still in my possession

but unknown to me
which I have not seen
nor disposed of
may it find common grave
with the dust of the earth ... '

(Gottlieb 1983, p. 129)

Having sought out *hametz* in the household—and within the members of the household—one is now concretely and intrapsychically prepared to enter the process of celebrating the experience of leaving enslavement by conducting the ritual of the Seder when evening arrives.

This process parallels that which Maidenbaum (1991, p. 300) identifies as central to Jung's consciously enunciated values, even while other destructive forces could grip him: 'I feel confident that this is what Jung himself would have approved of—the search for truth, for conscious and unconscious realities.'

Yachatz—Breaking and Splitting Off

The Passover Seder begins with the rituals of blessing and lighting candles, and blessing and partaking of wine (which serve to initiate all Jewish festivals) and a blessing over a spring vegetable, which is dipped in salt water and eaten.[7] These are followed by the first consternating actions of the Seder. A person at the table selects the middle of the three pieces of *matzah* that are stacked on a plate. Without a blessing, this person breaks the middle *matzah* into two pieces, one larger than the other. The larger piece is placed in a cloth and set aside; it will be used for the *afikomen* (from the Greek for dessert, that which comes after) which is required to be eaten at the conclusion of the meal, before the second half of the Seder can proceed. The smaller piece is returned to the middle position, between the two remaining pieces of *matzah*, both whole. The action of breaking that constitutes *Yachatz* activates the beating heart of the Seder: *Maggid*.

Maggid—What Needs To Be Told

Questions, which are very specific and embodied, pertaining to what is happening at the moment, inaugurate the process of *Maggid*, the telling:

What makes this night different from all other nights?
On all other nights we eat either leavened bread or matzah; on this night only matzah.
On all other nights we eat herbs of any kind; on this night only bitter herbs.
On all other nights we do not dip even once; on this night we dip twice.
On all other nights we eat our meal either sitting or reclining; on this night we all recline.

(Goldberg 2019, pp. 8–9)

What follows as an 'answer' is a story told in a rambling and disjointed manner, with detours and extremely detailed discussion. This telling begins with what seems to be a non-sequitur:

We were slaves of Pharaoh in Egypt and the Eternal One brought us out from there with a strong hand and an outstretched arm. Now if God had not brought out our ancestors from Egypt, then even we, our children, and our children's children might still have been enslaved to Pharaoh in Egypt. Therefore, even if we were all wise, all people of understanding, and even if we were all old and well-learned in the Torah, it would still be our duty to tell the story of the departure from Egypt. And the more one tells of the departure from Egypt, the more is one to be praised.

(Goldberg 2019, p. 9)

The telling of a story appears to have begun, even if it seems to have no relationship to the questions that were asked. But the apparent story is immediately interrupted by the description of a discussion that a group of rabbis had in the first century CE, centuries after that nascent story ostensibly would have taken place:

It happened that Rabbi Eliezer, Rabbi Joshua, Rabbi Elazar son of Azaria, Rabbi Akiba and Rabbi Tarfon reclined in B'nei Brak telling the story of the exodus from Egypt for the entire night, until their students came and said to them: Our Rabbis, the time has arrived to recite the morning prayers.

(Goldberg 2019, pp. 9–10)

On one level this story echoes and celebrates the value of dwelling on the story of escaping enslavement, as just announced in the *Haggadah*. However, there is also traditional commentary that understands this story in its social context: These same rabbis lived and taught in the era of the emperor Hadrian, who had forbidden Jews to gather, on pain of death, because of their subversive activity against Roman occupation. The Seder conducted here was not only a banned religious activity, but also a meeting to strategize their resistance to Roman rule. The students' alert to their teachers was a coded message that they needed to disband to avoid discovery by the approaching Romans. Attending to the foundation myth of liberation from Egypt engenders another form of liberation, revolution, and renewal. This is the core of the 'story' that needs to be told, the text that requires study.[8] Everything else is commentary.

The circuitous telling continues, dwelling and elaborating on details of the narrative. How did we become enslaved? What was slavery like? How did we get out of it? Passages are considered, detailing how the enslaved people came to register the suffering of enslavement and their outcry, as well as God's response to hearing this outcry. The ten plagues that afflicted the Egyptians before Pharaoh acceded to the demand that the Israelites be set free, are enumerated. Gratitude is offered for other events that occur later in the Biblical narrative.

Items on the ritual Seder plate, serving as props engaging different physical senses and qualities, are lifted up in turn and their significance is discussed, evoking experiences both of being enslaved and of leaving slavery.

The telling concludes with this statement: 'In every generation, each person is obligated to regard themselves as having personally left Egypt'.

The Seder continues after *Maggid* with psalms of praise, a second blessing over wine, washing hands, and blessing and consuming *matzah*, bitter herbs, and charoset. At this point, an intermission occurs in which dinner is served.

Tzafun—What Is Hidden

After the evening meal of the Seder has been enjoyed, the broken piece re-appears. It is customary for a form of serious play to ensue. One version is that the leader of the Seder has hidden the *afikomen* after setting it aside, and that now the children at the Seder are to search for it. Sharon Anisfeld, a contemporary woman rabbi, describes the moment this way:

> ... We lift the middle matzah and break it in two.
> The larger piece is hidden.
> To remind us that more is concealed than revealed. To remind us how much we do not know.
> How much we do not see.
> How much we have yet to understand.
>
> The larger piece is hidden and wrapped in a napkin.
> This is the *afikomen*.
> It will be up to the youngest to find it before the Seder can come to an end.
> (Anisfeld 2006, p. 56)

Another custom is that the children "steal" the *afikomen* and hold it for a ransom. Either way, the children inhabit a position of power, because the

Seder cannot continue until all the participants have eaten a piece of the *afikomen*. In Anisfeld's imagination:

> In this game of hide and seek,
> We remind ourselves that we do not begin to know all that our children
>
> will reveal to us.
> We do not begin to understand the mysteries they will uncover,
>
> The broken pieces they will find,
> The hidden fragments in need of repair ... '
>
> (Anisfeld 2006, p. 57)

Only when that negotiation has been successfully carried out can the Seder continue, with the blessings of gratitude to the transcendent one who is the ultimate source of all nourishment, including the meal that had just been concluded with the eating of the *afikomen*. The final sections of the Seder include two more blessings over wine, before and after psalms of praise to God, and songs that literally and metaphorically recount a variety of experiences of oppression and liberation from those oppressions. The Seder ends with the words 'Next year in Jerusalem', a longing for a future time and experience of un-dividedness, of inclusiveness, in the 'City of Wholeness'.[9]

Reparations

Carter spelled out the details of the reparations that he called for from the IAAP (Carter 2021). The white analysts of the JPA have our own continued reparations to make. I do not presume to name for those harmed what other reparations would adequately address the harm. However, I imagine that whatever the reparations need to be, they will involve—as in *bedikat hametz*—a recurring examination and intentional searching out of where the *hametz* of white privilege and puffed-up space-taking exist, acknowledging and eliminating it when we recognize it, and by doing so making more space available for other possibilities and other voices at the table. As a community what, as in *Yachatz*, have we split off and set aside? As in *Maggid*, this requires us to ask questions, be inquisitive about—and invite the telling of—the stories of exclusion, minimization and other harm that have not been told, that we have not heard, or that need to be told again, in great detail. As in overseeing the process of making *matzah*, the care and attention that we give to this process, and, the timeframe in which we carry out what is required, determine whether the outcome is life-giving, or, cuts us off from inner and outer connectedness and potential greater wholeness.

What is given in exchange for the *afikomen* is not a gift. Reparations also are not a gift; they are a debt that is owed, and that needs to be paid, for a life-giving process to continue in which we act on our purpose as a community of responsible analysts. Allowing the anxiety that we will not create a perfect written or spoken statement, whether on the level of an international psychoanalytic organization, regional institute, or individual writing in a book like this, and the fear of the mortification of causing more harm, can paralyze us on all levels, a resistance born of white fragility and psychoanalytic innocence (Sheehi 2021).

Transgression

Generally, children are not encouraged to steal and manipulate or force their parents or other adults into giving them what they demand. Yet the ritual of the Seder *requires* this transgressive act. In this moment, those who generally are outside of the sphere of power stand at its center.[10] The adults withdraw some of their customary authority (right to tell or direct the story and action) and there is space for children to voice their wishes and desires.

The negotiation over the redemption of the *afikomen* can engender anxiety: what will the demands be? How difficult will it be to meet them? What price will it entail? The negotiation can also be playful, in which there is a sense of aliveness and surprise. In this way, the theatre/play of the negotiations around the *afikomen* reflects the opening up of a transitional space (Winnicott 1971), which is safe because it is both contained *and* not full. There is room for discovery and imagination in the containing presence of a trusted other; there is space to think and imagine different possibilities and perspectives. The transcendent function can be constellated in this kind of space, a bridging connection between ego and self that may allow something authentic and new to come into being.

The process involves a sense of careful comprehensiveness and a sense of urgency. Like the rabbis simultaneously celebrating Passover and planning revolution, whose Seder must both dwell on the details necessary to feel the nature of the oppression and to discern paths to liberation, and still be concluded before mourning and discovery by the opposing forces. The negotiation must be successfully accomplished for the process to continue. There is the danger of further psychic harm when reparations, such as those Carter identified (2021), are not carried out in a timely fashion.

As the *Haggadah* calls for each person participating in the Seder to see themselves as having personally left Egypt, each of us in the psychoanalytic community must see ourself as personally involved in the process of addressing racism. If not, we will continue to harm others and be enslaved by our individual racism and the racism present in our foundational writings and theory. We express our hope in an ongoing commitment to attempt to prevent racist harm from continuing in our work as analysts, as an institute and as a psychoanalytic community.

We also register despair in the face of the inevitability that we as individuals and our psychoanalytic field will inflict racist harm in the future.

Reparative Transgression in our Community

Like the timeframe that requires the Seder to conclude by midnight, and the ransom of the *afikomen* substantially before then, there is an urgency in the need for a response to the call for such correctives, whenever they arise. I suggest that an attitude of serious play, like the negotiations for the *afikomen* in *Tzafun*, is called for in our psychoanalytic communities at such times. Such an attitude may burn away the inflated, puffed-up sense of importance and fragility, that is the *hametz* we must rid ourselves of, to make space at the table for what, and *who*, belongs there but has been excluded. This calls for a humility and grounded-ness, a *matzah* attitude, an embracing reconnection to the fundamentals of the best of psychoanalytic work, carefully observed and carried out.

The Book of Exodus specifies that when the Hebrews fled slavery in Egypt, the Egyptians gave them gifts. Jacob comments that, "The silver and gold given (not lent) by the Egyptians constituted protest against the policies of the royal tyrant. They demonstrated a renewal of public conscience" (Jacob 2001, p. 387). In addition to being a debt that we have a responsibility to pay, reparations are also a way to demonstrate a shift on a collective and cultural level. This collection of essays is one contribution to such protest and renewal of public conscience in the psychoanalytic sphere, even if the details necessarily are dated long before publication.

If the demands of reparations are met, what follows? In *Tzafun*, everyone participating is required to ingest and incorporate the *afikomen*. It is not pleasing and delicious (as the dessert that preceded it was); in the work of our psychoanalytic community, it is the flat, hard, unappealing reality of reckoning with the existence of racism in our field and of our personal implication in systemic racism, and the harm they have caused and continue to cause. It is dry in our mouths and hard to chew, and we must take it in. Otherwise, we must face what would be the *greater* price of having it remain split off into shadow, broken off from consciousness and responsibility, preventing any further development that would be engendered by genuine inclusiveness.

Although this is not, and cannot, be the intention of such reparations, another outcome could be that the JPA as a community becomes more capable *overall* of engendering a transitional space in which new voices and imaginations can be recognized and valued. The unintended but nonetheless real inhibitions—the narrow places—that have limited our community in the past might also shift more if we as a community become more aware of what individuals, as well as any creative theoretical and clinical possibilities, we have unconsciously, and even consciously, split off. We can choose to intentionally search for them, re-incorporate them, and invite them to make their demands upon us, transgressive as they may seem.

By making these choices, we have the opportunity to engage in reparative transgression, to commit ourselves to a process to repair, as much as possible, the harm that has been caused by who and what has been split off, and never made space for in our psychoanalytic community. Doing so involves crossing several boundaries: from unawareness to awareness; from space-occupying to space-making; from defensive protection of the past authorities to openness to new voices, those who will live with the consequences of what we have—and have not—reckoned with what reparations we have—and have not—made.

It is this state of being that is sought in engaging in the rituals of Passover, and a dynamic undergirding what we are seeking as a psychoanalytic community. A state in which differences have been constellated and can be held in conscious relationship with each other, with conflict, but without annihilation. It is a state in which we are not unconsciously enacting the role of either the oppressed or the oppressor, but one which constellates the energy that honors the capacity and right for each of us to be visible, to be heard, to be multi-dimensional rather than one-sided, to develop into more whole individuals and into a more whole community. The challenge to do so raises our greatest fears and our greatest hopes, and, is ultimately the only path consistent with the continued enlargement of our individual psyches and our psychoanalytic community. We have an ethical imperative to engage in the unending challenge of seeking out our personal racism and the racism of the psychoanalytic communities we are part of, in whatever forms they take, despite the mortification that doing so inevitably induces.

To the extent that anxiety about speaking freely in the community haunts the JPA in general, and regarding speaking about racism in our psychoanalytic tradition in particular, it inhibits what otherwise might be a freer, fuller, more individuated process within community. It keeps us as a psychoanalytic community in a narrow place, an Egypt that confines us to what has been, not the fuller version of what we can be.

In this spirit, we can take up with meaning the challenge and paradox of reparative transgressions. We can continue to seek out the *hametz* of our own racism and that of our field, and we can continue to seek out our fear of speaking about what we find, naming it when we come across it. Performing this kind of careful observation, we can provide the central form of sustenance necessary for our community, as the ingredients of *matzah* are attended to for Passover. In doing so, we avoid psychological and communal *karet*, radical isolation from relationship with others and with the otherness that abides within us. Instead, like eating the *afikomen*, if we can take up, with meaning, the paradox of reparative transgressions, we integrate—we consciously take back into ourselves, the shadow element of our racism, acknowledging that which had been ruptured, split off and hidden from conscious awareness. We must do this in order to continue with the process of celebrating whatever freedom we may have. Our freedom comes at the cost of others, known or unknown to us.

It is not our task to complete this work, and we are not free to neglect it. As analysts, we have an ethical imperative to continue to reckon with racism in ourselves and our analytic community; to observe it, revisit it, to elaborate on it, to hear the story that needs to be told, to ask questions that are not rote but responsive to what is before us, to seek out what harm we have inflicted and been unconscious of, to ask those we have harmed what they would experience as reparative and to provide it, and, to rework this process regularly, bearing the anxiety and mortification required in crossing into the territories involved.

The Seder ends with yearning. This closing statement is paradoxically an acknowledgement of the eternal incompleteness of the process of collective psychological and concrete freedom *and* an assertion of that possibility. As bell hooks recognizes:

> There are times when personal experience keeps us from reaching the mountain top and so we let it go because the weight of it is too heavy. And sometimes the mountain top is difficult to reach with all our resources, factual and confessional, so we are just there, collectively grasping, feeling the limitations of knowledge, longing together, yearning for a way to reach that highest point. Even this yearning is a way to know.
>
> (hooks 1994, p. 44)

Notes

1 Although I have named Black and Brown analysands, candidates and analysts, the same challenge applies to all people of color, Native Peoples, members of queer, non-binary, transgender or any communities othered in our society, which privileges white, European-descended, male, cis-gender and heterosexual members.
2 Ann Ulanov, verbal communication.
3 By writing this, I do not intend either to congratulate or to denigrate myself or the group; I intend to describe a process that feels both necessary and inadequate if I am to follow the ethical imperative of our field.
4 It may be that my peripheral relationship to the JPA for many years led these analysts and candidates to feel free to communicate this kind of experience to me.
5 There is no convincing archaeological or historical evidence that the Exodus from Egypt occurred.
6 Here I use 'them' as an inclusive pronoun; the original text of the Haggadah reads 'he'.
7 Although blessing a vegetable before eating it is a traditional act in Judaism, dipping a food in another substance is a custom borrowed from the symposium. Saltwater in particular often is understood in part as a reference to tears shed in the suffering of slavery.
8 Rabbi Akiba, one of the quintet of subversive rabbis, was also known for asserting to the teachers and students of the ancient House of Study that study is great because it leads to action.
9 I recognize that the Israeli occupation of Palestine, including Jerusalem, is itself an example of brutally racist harm. I do not suggest that Jewish people have a claim on Jerusalem; rather, I note this as an expression of an archetypal longing for wholeness, and appreciate that this longing itself without awareness of its shadow is destructive.

10 By this I do not intend to suggest that Black and Brown candidates, analysts, or lay people are 'childish' or 'childlike'; rather, that their (intentional or unintentional) exclusion by white members and leaders, who have inhabited all the space, and their subsequent absence from a meaningful place at the table, has resulted in a situation in which they have not had full recognition for influence and voice, *as if* they were not 'adults' with a place at the table.

References

Adams, M.V. (1996). *The Multi-Cultural Imagination: 'Race', Colour and the Unconscious.* London: Routledge.

Anisfeld, S. (2006). 'How Much We Have Yet to Understand.' In *The Women's Seder Sourcebook*, eds.S. Anisfeld, T. Mohr & C. Spector (pp. 56–57). Woodstock: Jewish Lights.

Cahan, L., ed. (1998). *Siddur Sim Shalom for Shabbat and Holidays.* New York: United Synagogue of Conservative Judaism.

Brewster, F. (2017). *African Americans and Jungian Psychology: Leaving the Shadows.* London & New York: Routledge.

Brewster, F. (2020). *The Racial Complex: A Jungian Perspective on Culture and Race.* London & New York: Routledge.

Brewster, F. & Morgan, H. (2022). *Racial Legacies: Jung, Politics and Culture.* London & New York: Routledge.

Carter, C.J. (2021). 'Time for Space at the Table: An African American/Native American Analyst-in-training's First-hand Reflections. A Call for the IAAP to Publicly Denounce (But Not Erase) the White Supremacist Writings of C.G. Jung'. *Journal of Analytical Psychology*, 66, 1, 70–92.

Darwall, S. (2006). *The Second-Person Standpoint: Morality, Respect and Accountability.* Cambridge, MA: Harvard University Press.

DiAngelo, R. (2018). *White Fragility: Why It's So Hard for White People to Talk About Racism.* Boston: Beacon Press.

Goldberg, N. (2019). *Passover Haggadah.* Brooklyn: KTAV Publishing House.

Gottlieb, L. (1983). 'Spring Cleaning Ritual on the Eve of Full Moon Nisan'. In *On Being a Jewish Feminist*, ed.S. Heschel. New York: Schocken Books.

hooks, b. (1994). *Teaching to Transgress: Education as the Practice of Freedom.* London: Routledge.

Jacob, B. (2001). Commentary in *Etz Hayim: Torah and Commentary.* Philadelphia: The Jewish Publication Society.

Jung, C.G. (1917/1972). 'Preface to the Second Edition'. *CW 7*. Princeton: Princeton University Press.

Kimbles, S. (2014). *Phantom Narratives: The Unseen Contributions of Culture to Psyche.* Maryland: Rowman & Littlefield.

Maidenbaum, A. (1991). 'Lingering Shadows: A Personal Perspective'. *Lingering Shadows: Jungians, Freudians and Anti-Semitism.* A. Maidenbaum & S. Martin, eds. Boston & London: Shambhala Publications.

Maidenbaum, A. & Martin, S., eds. (1991). *Lingering Shadows: Jungians, Freudians and Anti-Semitism.* Boston & London: Shambhala Publications.

Morgan, H. (2021). *The Work of Whiteness: A Psychoanalytic Perspective*. London: Routledge.

Rothberg, M. (2019). *The Implicated Subject: Beyond Victims and Perpetrators*. Stanford: Stanford University Press.

Sheehi, L. & Sheehi, S. (2021). *Psychoanalysis Under Occupation: Practicing Resistance in Palestine*. London: Routledge.

Winnicott, D.W. (1971). *Playing and Reality*. London: Tavistock Publications Limited.

Zornberg, A.G. (2001). *The Particulars of Rapture: Reflections on Exodus*. New York: Doubleday.

Index

For Product Safety Concerns and Information please contact our EU
representative GPSR@taylorandfrancis.com Taylor & Francis Verlag GmbH,
Kaufingerstraße 24, 80331 München, Germany

Printed and bound by CPI Group (UK) Ltd, Croydon, CR0 4YY
08/06/2025
01897006-0017